The Maudsley Handbook of Practical Psychiatry

Third Edition

Edited by

DAVID GOLDBERG
Director of Medical Education
The Bethlem Maudsley NHS Trust
London, UK

Oxford   New York   Tokyo
OXFORD UNIVERSITY PRESS
1997

Oxford University Press, Great Clarendon Street, Oxford OX2 6DP

Oxford   New York

Athens   Auckland   Bangkok   Bogota   Bombay   Buenos Aires
Calcutta   Cape Town   Dar es Salaam   Delhi   Florence   Hong Kong
Istanbul   Karachi   Kuala Lumpur   Madras   Madrid   Melbourne
Mexico City   Nairobi   Paris   Singapore   Taipei   Tokyo   Toronto
and associated companies in
Berlin   Ibadan

Oxford is a trade mark of Oxford University Press

Published in the United States
by Oxford University Press Inc., New York

A catalogue record for this book is available from the British Library

Library of Congress Cataloging in Publication Data
(Data available)

ISBN 0 19 262853 4 plb

Printed in Great Britain by
The Bath Press, Bath

Preface

This edition of the *Maudsley 'Orange Book'* represents a break with tradition. Instead of this manual being written by teachers for trainees, containing only those things which we thought essential for them, this edition has been planned by the trainees themselves. As a result, many sections now make their appearance for the first time. The Maudsley Junior Common Room appointed five of its members to a working party, and this met three times with the Editor to decide what should go into the book. The book contains advice on managing difficult interview situations, as well as up-to-date advice about early treatment — which should be invaluable for young psychiatrists on duty. The recommendations of the 1993 Code of Practice are of increasing importance, and we have summarized some of the more important points from this, as well as including guidance on the Care Programme Approach, Needs Assessment, and the Supervision Register.

In some cases, our decision was that the text should be written by an experienced teacher: we have Dinesh Bhugra, Alec Buchanan, Lachlan Campbell, Stuart Checkley, Michael Crowe, Sue Davidson, David Goldberg, John Gunn, Frank Holloway, Rob Kerwin, Channi Kumar, Anthony Mann, Jane Marshall, Clive Meux, Mike Philpot, George Szmukler, Maria Ron, Eric Taylor, Brian Toone, Janet Treasure, and Simon Wessely to thank for relevant parts of the text.

However, much was written by the trainees themselves: Kam Bhui, Jonathon Bindman, Wai Chen, Paul Cotter, Helen Crimlisk, Emily Finch, Nick Glozier, Louise Howard, Philip Lucas, Jan Neeleman, Celia Taylor, Mark Taylor, Sarah Welch, Roger Weissman, and Ben Wright all contributed.

We have tried to write a textbook that will help trainees everywhere. Our sections on the 'When to refer' chapter inevitably assume that a wide range of specialist services are available, obviously these must be modified in places where this is not the case. As Editor, I take responsibility for what follows.

The Maudsley Hospital   D. G.
February 1997

Acknowledgement

The ICD-10 Classification of Mental and Behavioural Disorders (Categories F00 through to F99) is reproduced with the kind permission of the World Health Organization.

Contents

Abbreviations

ADL	activities of daily living
AMTS	Abbreviated Mental Test Score
APA	American Psychiatric Society
AST	aspartate aminotransferase (serum)
ASW	approved social worker
AUDIT	Alcohol Use Disorders Identification Test
BNF	British National Formulary
BPRS	Brief Psychiatric Rating Scale
BPS	British Psychological Society
CAGE	Cut (down) …Annoyed…Guilty…Eye (opener) (drinking problem)
CAN	Camberwell Assessment of Needs
CDT	carbohydrate-deficient transferrin
CNS	central nervous system
CPA	Care Programme Approach
CPK	creatinine phosphokinase
CPN	community psychiatric nurse
CSA	child sexual abuse
CSF	cerebrospinal fluid
CT	computed tomography
CVA	cerebrovascular accident
CXR	chest X-ray
CYP2D6	cytochrome oxidase enzyme 2PD6
DSH	deliberate self-harm
DSMIV	Diagnostic and Statistical Manual
DTF	Drug Tariff Formula
DTs	delirium tremens
ECG	electrocardiogram
ECT	electroconvulsive therapy
EEG	electroencephalogram
EPSE	extrapyrimidal side-effects
ESR	erythrocyte sedimentation rate
ESRS	Extra pyramidal symptoms rating scale
GABA	gamma-aminobutyric acid

GGT	gamma-glutamyltransferase
HIV	human immunodeficiency virus
ICD-10	International Classification of Diseases — 10th edn
ICU	intensive care unit
IgG	immunoglobulin G
IM	intramuscular
IV	intravenous
LSD	lysergic acid diethylamide
LTM	long-term memory
LUNSERS	Liverpool University side effect rating scale
MAOI	monoamine oxidase inhibitor
MAST	Michigan Alcoholism Screening Test
MCV	mean corpuscular volume
MDMA	methylene dioxy methamphetamine
MHRT	Mental Health Review Tribunal
MMSE	Mini-mental State Examination
MND	motor neurone disease
MRI	magnetic resonance imaging
MS	multiple sclerosis
MSE	mental state examination
NHS	National Health Service
NMS	neuroleptic malignant syndrome
OCP	oral contracepive pill
PANSS	Positive and negative symptom scale
PD	Parkinson's disease
PET	positron emission tomography
RMO	responsible medical officer
SD	supervised discharged
SLE	systemic lupus erythematosus
SPECT	single photon emission computed tomography (also known as SPET)
SR	Supervision register
SSRI	selective serotonin reuptake inhibitor
STM	short-term memory
TCA	tricyclic antidepressant
TFT	thyroid function test
TPHA	*Treponema pallidum* haemagglutination (test)

TPR	temperature, pulse, and respiration
VDRL	Venereal Disease Research Laboratory (test)
WHO	World Health Organization

1
The psychiatric interview with adults

This chapter distinguishes between the different interview techniques used when making a full assessment of a patient (see below) and those required while on emergency duty (p. 14). There are special considerations when interviewing elderly patients (p. 14) or those with learning disability (p. 18).

Interviews on the ward or out-patient department

Recording information elicited from the interview

Notes are best written at the time of the interview, remembering to name and date each sheet and to give the time of the interview on the first sheet; it is rare that the busy clinician will have time to write up notes after meetings. Some doctors find it helpful to record information under different headings on several sheets at once, this is particularly useful when recording verbatim examples of speech for the mental state examination.

The general structure of the interview

The interview process can be split into 'joining' with the patient and **establishing trust**: this provides the basis for the **assessment** which is an iterative process of information acquisition, hypothesis generation, and further information acquisition. The third stage of the interview is more therapeutic in emphasis and consists of education, forming the **management plan** with the patient, and communicating it to them. The final stage of the interview consists of **terminating** the interview.

The start of the interview and 'joining' with the patient

After introducing yourself, explain who you are and why you wish to see the patient. If relatives are present ask them if there is anything they feel you should know about before seeing the patient and explain that they will have an opportunity to speak to you after the interview. Generally, it is best to see adult patients alone.

In the interview room, reintroduce yourself to the patient (many will forget or mishear your name, and you will want to use this as part of your cognitive assessment later), then explain the purpose of the interview. Explain that you need to write some notes, but say that they are a confidential record. However, if the assessment is for medico-legal purposes it should be clearly stated that what is said in the interview will be put in a report which may be given to third parties or placed before the court. In this situation the patient should be asked to give written consent. Say how much time you expect to have available. Generally, it is advisable to avoid lengthy interviews and it is best to collect information over a number of days.

The assessment phase: the interview

The first areas to be addressed in any assessment are the presenting complaints and their history. Having elicited the history of the presenting complaint(s) it is often then most useful to make an assessment of the patient's mental state (see Chapter 4); this will complete your assessment of the present problem and put you in a better position for deciding how much detail you are going to need about the aetiology of the problem, the factors that precipitated the present crisis, and those that are maintaining it. The remainder of the assessment interview should be conducted with this in mind. Focus in depth on areas of interest, but obtain key information for less important areas which may be addressed at a later stage either at the end of the interview, if there is sufficient time, or on a later occasion. Detailed guidance for taking a history is given below (see pp. 4–11).

Forming a management plan

It may be necessary to complete your information gathering from other sources before proceeding to this stage of the assessment. If a relative is available, ask the patient whether they mind if you see them. (A parent of a child under 16 years of age has a legal right to see you, but patients over the age of 16 can object.) Use your judgement about whether to have the relative in the room while the management plan is communicated to the patient. Other things being equal, this is usually preferable, as the relative's attitude to what you propose is likely to be a critical factor in determining compliance, and the patient may not remember everything that you say.

Ask the patient how they expected you would help them. If their expectations sound reasonable, give them details of what you think would be the best course, and ask them whether that sounds reasonable to them.

If their expectations are quite different from your own, explain your reasons for preferring a different course of action. The relative is often very useful at this point, if they are present. Give your advice simply and clearly, bit by bit, and get the patient to agree with what you are saying.

If the patient needs an **investigation**, explain why, what it will involve, and what steps the patient needs to take to get it done. If you are referring the patient to a colleague, tell them your colleague's name and the reason for the referral.

If you are **prescribing a drug**, say: 'The drug I usually use for your problem is (name of the drug). Have you heard of that?' (If they have, have they ever been prescribed it, and did it help?) Tell them:

- the main effects of the drug
- its side-effects
- how long they are likely to have to take it
- and whether it is habit-forming.

If you are suggesting a **course of therapeutic interviews**, say:

- how many interviews you propose, and how long each will last
- what the purpose of the interviews will be
- what you expect the patient to discuss during them.

Get the patient to agree to the plan, or you may well waste your time.

Termination of the interview

Tell the patient what you are going to do — for example, write to their doctor, discuss their case with a colleague — and when they should hear from the hospital, or, in the case of in-patients, when they will next see you. You may not know exactly when you will be available to see a ward patient — but do give them some idea; for instance, 'I'm next here on Thursday, and I'll try to see you for half-an-hour during the afternoon'. If they are seen as out-patients, give them an appointment card with an identifying number on it. If you expect the patient to do anything, make sure this has been clearly understood by either the patient or their relative.

History of presenting complaint

Do not start writing until you have established the order in which the various complaints developed. Write an account in chronological order, giving the duration of each complaint or problem. This account of the evolution of the patient's problems should include the social milieu within which the symptoms developed, highlighting any key precipitating events. The patient's symptoms, attributions, and understanding of their experience should be described, as well as how he tried to cope with his experience.

The effects of any treatment taken should be noted. The effect of the patient's symptoms on his social, occupational, interpersonal (family, marriage, sexual functioning, responsibility) functioning and self-care (including eating, sleeping, weight, excretory functions, and substance use), should be described. Finally, recapitulate this history back to the patient, ask: 'Is that right?', and: 'Is there anything else?' At this stage go on to the mental state examination (p. 77).

Certain topics may come up during the history, including those described below.

Suicidal thoughts and actions

The questions form a natural hierarchy, which one goes along with as far as necessary:

• Do you feel that you have a future?

- Do you feel that life's not worth living?
- Do you ever feel completely hopeless?
- Do you ever feel you'd be better off dead and away from it all?
- Have you made any plans? (If overdose: have you handled the tablets?)
- Have you ever made an attempt to take your own life?
- What prevents you doing it?
- Have you made any arrangements for your affairs after your death?

After an episode of deliberate self-harm

Ask about: previous suicide attempts; current life problems, including trouble with finances or the law; history of alcohol and/or drug abuse/dependence; epilepsy; current poor physical health.

Eating disorders

- Do you think you have problems with your weight and eating?
- Are your doctors or any of your family and friends concerned about your weight and eating?
- Do you ever have times where you feel that your eating is out of control and so you quickly eat an enormous amount of food, much more than anyone else you know?

Epilepsy

- Do you suffer from epileptic attacks/blackouts?
- Has any doctor made a diagnosis of epilepsy?
- Do you take (should you take) drugs for treatment of epilepsy?

Life charts

It is often helpful to relate events in the patient's life to previous illnesses. Life charts are especially valuable if the patient has both a physical illness and psychological problems — the columns should then be: age; life event; physical illness; psychological illness. The 'physical illness' column may, of course, be omitted if there is nothing to record.

In its simplest form, there is a line for each year of the patient's life; but it may be more informative to use a non-linear time scale, giving more space to some key periods of the patient's life and less to others.

Family history

The amount of detail recorded will be influenced by the nature of the patient's illness. It is very helpful to draw a picture of the patient's family, using squares for males and circles for females. For siblings, enter their first name against the appropriate symbol. Deceased relatives are indicated by an oblique line through the circle or square, together with the date and cause of death. Marriages ended by divorce are indicated by a double oblique line. For example, see Fig. 1.1.

Draw this figure with the patient's assistance, and in full view. Then ask: 'Did anyone in your family suffer from a mental illness?'; if so, enter details against them. This is the most informative way of collecting information about genetic loading.

Personal history

In addition to collecting facts, use this opportunity to collect information about the patient's life which may help you to understand the presenting problems. Test hypotheses about the patient, using a 'negotiating' style: 'I wonder whether....'

Childhood

Place of birth and birth difficulties. Who brought the patient up and where: occupation of parents or care-giver, general nature and quality of relationship with each?

Family atmosphere
General experience of being a child in that family, were they happy times? (if not, what was the problem?). Early childhood difficulties and general development. (See also p. 49, Chapter 3.)

School
Age at leaving school and qualifications obtained. How did the patient get on with teachers and other students? What were the patient's best subjects?

Occupational history

Age at first job, general areas of employment, periods of unemployment and why. Frequency of job change. Current job, enjoyable, any problems? (This provides an opportunity to judge whether the patient has realized his or her potential; whether the patient has persistence. Frequent changes of job or leaving many jobs without good reason suggest an abnormal personality.)

Psychosexual history

Current 'partner': time with that person; difficulties; supportive? Previous partners. Age at first girl/boyfriend (ask directly about both same and opposite sexual relationships). Age at puberty and first sexual experience. Any unwanted sexual experiences? Any unsafe sex? If patient has steady partner, ask about the relationship. Any children (details)? (See p. 153 for fuller details.)

Past psychiatric history

Illnesses, admissions, treatment, and episodes of self-harm.

Past medical and surgical history

Full details of any illnesses.

Medication

Current medication. Any allergies or problems with medication.

Illustrative family tree

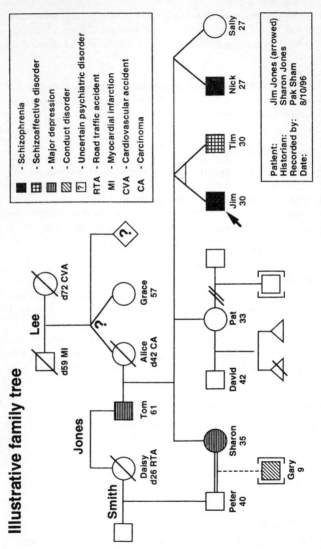

■	- Schizophrenia
⊞	- Schizoaffective disorder
▥	- Major depression
▨	- Conduct disorder
?	- Uncertain psychiatric disorder
RTA	- Road traffic accident
MI	- Myocardial infarction
CVA	- Cardiovascular accident
CA	- Carcinoma

Patient: Jim Jones (arrowed)
Historian: Sharon Jones
Recorded by: Pak Sham
Date: 8/10/96

Fig. 1.1

List of symbols used in family trees

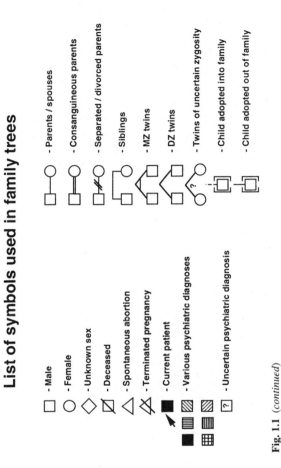

- Male
- Female
- Unknown sex
- Deceased
- Spontaneous abortion
- Terminated pregnancy
- Current patient
- Various psychiatric diagnoses
- Uncertain psychiatric diagnosis

- Parents / spouses
- Consanguineous parents
- Separated / divorced parents
- Siblings
- MZ twins
- DZ twins
- Twins of uncertain zygosity
- Child adopted into family
- Child adopted out of family

Fig. 1.1 (*continued*)

Alcohol use

All patients should be asked about their alcohol consumption. Screening aims to detect whether an alcohol problem is present, and, if so, whether it is likely to respond to brief intervention or to require specialized treatment. There are two main methods of screening: (1) questionnaires/interview; (2) biochemical and haematological markers. The first method is rapid, non-invasive, and inexpensive, but depends on the truthfulness of the patient. Laboratory tests such as gamma-glutamyltransferase (GGT), mean corpuscular volume (MCV), and serum aspartate aminotransferase (AST) may be helpful if the patient does not admit to heavy or problem drinking. These tests are less sensitive and more costly than questionnaires and are possibly best reserved for medical settings. Newer methods such as carbohydrate-deficient transferrin (CDT) show initial promise.

A number of screening questionnaires are available, including the Michigan Alcoholism Screening Test (MAST); the CAGE questionnaire and the Alcohol Use Disorders Identification Test (AUDIT). The MAST was developed to detect severe alcohol problems. The CAGE questionnaire widely used in primary care is helpful in identifying concerns about drinking:

Have you ever felt you should **C**ut down on your drinking?
Have people **A**nnoyed you by criticizing your drinking?
Have you ever felt bad or **G**uilty about your drinking?
Have you ever had a drink first thing in the morning to steady your nerves or to get rid of a hangover (**E**ye opener)?

The AUDIT aims to identify harmful drinking at an early stage, but it can also detect alcohol dependence (see Appendix 6 for the full AUDIT). It comprises 10 items which can be administered by non-clinical workers or be self-administered. The items cover alcohol consumption, symptoms of alcohol use, and consequences of alcohol use. Screening with the AUDIT can be carried out in a variety of primary care and community settings. The core questions:

- How often do you have a drink containing alcohol?
- How many drinks containing alcohol do you have on a typical day when you are drinking?

- How often do you have six or more drinks on one occasion?

can be made less threatening by being incorporated into an assessment of general health/lifestyle or into the medical history. See also pp. 146–9.

Drug misuse

All patients should be asked about their use of illicit or over-the-counter drugs. However, for most patients a few brief screening questions will suffice; for example:

- Are there any other tablets or medicines that you take, apart from those you get from your doctor?
- Is there anything you buy from the chemists, or get from friends?
- Have you used any (illegal) drugs such as ... amphetamines/ speed, ecstasy, cocaine/crack, LSD/acid, or heroin?
- What about tablets to settle your nerves or to help you sleep (such as temazepam or diazepam)? See also pp. 149–52.

Forensic history

Have you ever been in trouble with the law or had points on your driving licence? If so, record full details.

Social history

Accommodation, finances, home activities, outside activities, carers. (For fuller details, see p. 58, Chapter 3.)

Personality

Before you became unwell what were you like? Prompt the patient for whether they had many friends; could they trust people; what their temper was like; how they coped with life; how they dealt with criticism; were they very tidy?

(Remember that information from an informant is much more valuable than that from the patient — the patient's views are usually influenced by the current illness. For more details, see p. 56.)

Interviews on emergency duty

The actual interview with the patient is always the kingpin of any psychiatric assessment, but it should not be forgotten that the interview will be affected by the preparation for and the setting of the interview itself. This, of course, is determined before the patient is seen. Preparation falls into obtaining background information and preparing the setting. The actual assessment made on emergency duty is likely to focus more on the presenting problem than the fuller assessments carried out on the wards.

Background information including the referral

Obtaining background information will enhance the efficiency and effectiveness of the assessment as well as promoting greater safety, but it does lay the clinician open to bias. In most situations, information is usually limited and in the form of a letter. Background information becomes particularly important in the context of the psychiatric emergency.

The commonest psychiatric examination the trainee will have to undertake is the emergency assessment in the hospital setting. Typically, the patient will be heralded by a telephone call. For each call, the following details should be elicited and clearly recorded in the notes, remembering that this may be the only opportunity to obtain some of the information:

The name of the referrer, who they are in relation to the patient, and how you can contact them again.

The patient's name and address (including postcode) and general details including the referrer's concerns.

At this stage, before accepting the referral, if you are in any doubt about whether or not the patient falls within your remit, explain this to the referring agent and arrange to call them back with the details (including telephone number) of the correct institution.

Then ask the referrer for details of why they wish to send this patient to you, both in terms of their concerns regarding the patient and how they feel that the patient should or might be helped. If the referral is a result of unusual behaviour record a detailed account of who observed what.

This is particularly important for patients who are brought by the police (for example, under a Section 136) as this may be the only objective, collaborative information available on the patient, and the only opportunity to elicit and record it.

Where the referrer is a health-care professional obtain as much information as possible. This can be grouped into:

- physical health problems (past and current, including medication)
- mental health problems (past, current assessment, and medication)
- risk to self, and
- risk to others (past and current).

Agree with the referrer where and when the patient will be seen.

Preparation of the interview room

The practical aspects of eliciting and recording information should be considered: quiet; well lit; private; with a writing surface. Typically, the optimal seating arrangement is at an angle of 45–90 degrees, for example around one corner of a desk. Safety issues must **always** be considered before seeing every patient, these include (see p. 131, Chapter 6):

- Never sit the patient between you and your exit from the room, or have any barrier between you and your exit (table or patient).
- Remove any object from sight that might be used as a weapon, for example letter openers or large paperweights. In a volatile situation the act of sighting a potential weapon can catalyse decompensation into violence.
- If there is a panic button in the room know where it is, how it works, and whether or not it will summon aid after hours. If there is no panic button know how to summon help.
- Avoid using rooms that are in an isolated area.
- Inform nursing colleagues what you are doing and how long you expect to be.

- If you believe that there is a more than usual safety risk then arrange for correspondingly greater numbers of (nursing) colleagues to be in increasing proximity. Before the interview discuss your concerns and how to manage an unwanted event.

Assessments on emergency duty

It would be inappropriate to attempt to cover all aspects of history-taking while on emergency duty. The work is of necessity problem-focused, dealing with only those aspects of the history and examination necessary for understanding the nature of the patient's present problems. Thus, the history of the present symptoms and a focused mental state examination are essential, as well as detailed enquiry about drugs and medications taken (or not taken) recently. Previous psychiatric history should be covered briefly, and an effort should be made to collect information from others who are accompanying the patient.

The doctor will wish to admit all those whose illness represents a threat either to themselves or others, unless satisfactory alternative care arrangements are available. Re-admissions of psychotic patients can sometimes be prevented if the keyworker is available, or if resources permit a very brief stay in a community hostel whilst medication is resumed.

Interviews with elderly patients

These are essentially the same as for younger adults, but there are differences of emphasis that need consideration. Assessment is frequently complicated by the patient's **intellectual impairment, physical ill-health** including hearing and visual disability, and **clouding of consciousness.** As a consequence it may be necessary to carry out the assessment over several sessions and it is essential to obtain a **collateral history** from a close relative or carer. Nowadays, the initial assessment will usually be carried out in the patient's own home.

Old-age psychiatry is largely concerned with four major diagnoses: dementia; delirium; depression; delusional disorder (including schizophrenia). Clearly, neuroses, personality disorders, and substance abuse do occur in the elderly, but to simplify what follows, discussion will be limited to the four diagnostic groups listed above.

History of presenting complaint

Bear in mind that some patients with dementia or delirium may lack insight. Also that direct questioning about memory function may be helpful:

- Do you have any difficulty with your memory?
- Do you forget where you have left things more than you used to?
- Do you think your memory is worse than other people of your age?

Other cognitive problems, such as dysphasia, dyspraxia, and agnosia should be asked about (see pp. 92–3).

Elderly patients may not admit to feeling 'depressed' or 'low in spirits', careful questioning as to other depressive symptoms, (for example, suicidal ideas, diurnal variation, low self-esteem, hopelessness, guilt, insomnia, and anorexia and weight loss), will assist in making the diagnosis.

Paranoid or psychotic features may need to be elicited directly:

- Do you get on well with your neighbours or have you had any difficulty with them?
- Do you ever hear/see things that other people do not? Are people spying on you or plotting against you?
- Are people stealing from you?

Many patients with dementia present to psychiatric services because of associated psychotic, affective, or behavioural disturbances, rather than the cognitive problems. **These are best elicited from an informant**.

Common psychotic symptoms in dementia include:

- delusions of theft, persecution
- auditory and visual hallucinations
- misidentification syndromes.

Common behavioural problems include:

- wandering
- aggression
- urinary incontinence
- elements of the Kluver–Bucy syndrome (that is to say, binge-eating, hyperorality, sexual disinhibition, misrecognition, rages, apathy, and hypermetamorphosis).

Ask whether symptoms were of sudden or gradual onset; the order in which symptoms developed is sometimes important, for instance in differentiating depression with cognitive impairment from 'real' dementia, and in differentiating between different types of dementia.

Family history

Specifically, a history in first-degree relatives of:

- dementia, Parkinson's disease, mental illness
- heart or stroke disease, hypertension
- cancer including leukaemia
- Down's syndrome.

Personal history

Academic level should be determined, since low attainment at school (Standard 6[1] or less) may indicate low premorbid intelligence. This may be a contributory factor to poor cognitive performance.

Enquire about traumatic experiences occurring during wartime (or at other times) which still bother the patient or cause distress.

Sexual activity should be asked about in a straightforward and direct way. It should not be assumed that sexual activity will have ceased simply because a person is old.

---

[1] Standard 6 was the penultimate grade at school prior to leaving at age 14.

Ask about reaction to life events:

- retirement
- bereavement
- serious illness in the patient or a close relative.

Elder abuse is being increasingly recognized. A neutral series of questions which may allow further exploration of this difficult area include:

- Has anyone shouted or insulted you recently?
- Has anyone hit you or handled you roughly recently?
- Has anyone stopped you getting the help you need recently?

Social history

This follows the usual schema outlined on p. 58; however important areas in the elderly, other than housing and finance, include:

- *Social network* — what support is there from family/friends, clubs; what day-centres are attended, how frequently?
- *Home-care support* — does the patient receive meals-on-wheels, home-helps, and district nurses; how frequently, are they helpful?

Lastly, an account of the patient's ability to perform activities of daily living (ADL) should be obtained. This should include information on the following:

- *Mobility* — the use of walking aids, can stairs be climbed without help.
- *Personal hygiene* — washing, continence, using the toilet, and dressing. (for example, 'Can you wash yourself without help? Do you have trouble controlling your bladder? Can you dress yourself without help?')
- *Domestic activities* — cooking, laundry, housework, and paying bills.

Interviews with patients with a learning disability

People with a mild learning disability can usually provide their own history; additional history from an informant will usually be needed when the patient is moderately or severely disabled.

Remember that learning disability is not in itself an emergency; it is a permanent condition. Learning disability does **not** protect against the development of other conditions.

Always obtain information on the nature and duration of any recent changes, particularly behavioural changes: the opportunity to obtain this information from a **key informant** may not arise again.

In a genuine emergency, usually some **additional condition** has developed: this may be either physical or mental.

- Always eliminate **pain** as a cause for an acute behavioural disturbance: pain may arise from a life-threatening condition.
- Ask about recent **seizures** or other epileptic phenomena.

If a diagnosis of learning disability is in doubt ask the informant:

- Was this person's development delayed in childhood?
- Did this person attend a Special School?
- Did they learn to read and write?
- What jobs has this person held?
- Is this person losing any skills?
- Does anyone in the family have a learning disability or developmental abnormality?

2
The psychiatric interview with children

Some differences from interviewing adults

- The child is *brought* — the reasons may not have been explained to them or they may be inaccurate. The child may believe he is going to be told off, taken away, kept, or hurt. They may be waiting for a blood test or operation.
- The child is not the main informant.
- The child may not answer any questions, no matter how experienced the psychiatrist. Sometimes children, or even teenagers, who will not speak can be persuaded to draw or play a game.
- The experience of *uninterrupted* time with total attention from a sympathetic adult will be new to many children.

Setting

The psychiatrist will already have introduced him- or herself to the child. With younger children the doctor should get down to the child's eyelevel by kneeling or squatting to ask them their name and how old they are. Care should be taken to acknowledge siblings who may be present.

There are great advantages in ensuring that diagnostic interviews with children of similar age are broadly comparable. The interview room should be arranged so that only the objects which the psychiatrist considers will be needed are in view. The toys and games which are available need to be chosen with care to facilitate those types of observations which are of greatest diagnostic value. Observation of a child is much more difficult in a room cluttered with toys. For the child aged 6 or more it is usually preferable to spend most of the interview talking with the child in the manner outlined below. With younger children and those with language or global delay there will need to be a greater reliance placed on non-verbal communication, and interaction will generally be easier if it occurs in a play situation.

With more mature children or adolescents the interview may often take more the form of the adult psychiatric interview, but considerable modifications are still required since adults often present because of their own concern over their problems. By contrast, the child or adolescent is generally referred because of someone else's concern.

Observe the parent–child interaction in the waiting room when collecting the child for interview. How do the parents handle the separation? How does the child respond? Are the parents warm, critical, hostile, detached, or understanding in the way they talk to the child?

General advice

- Be non-judgemental.
- Be prepared to specify limits — destruction and rage are not cathartic. 'That's not what people do here,' 'I want you to stop doing that'.
- Avoid long silences which can become persecutory, particularly for adolescents — some can be engaged in a game, some will respond to 'I wonder if …'.
- Accept pictures if offered, and keep them safe, because they will be asked about another time. Pictures should not be put in the place of honour on the wall, it will be impossible to do this for all the children who come and someone else may take them down.
- Do not speak in an artificial voice — children are quite tone responsive.
- Do not rush in with direct interpretations.
- Do not let the child take toys out of the room. 'Sorry, these toys belong to the hospital and there would be none for you to play with if you took one home every time.'
- Warn about the end of the session 5 minutes before it finishes.

Common errors

Beware the pitfalls of:

- keeping off relevant, but difficult topics in pursuit of a pleasant experience for the child;
- siding with the child instead of displaying a constructive neutrality;
- leading a suggestible child into inappropriate answers;
- 'building castles in the air' on the nods of mute children.

Engagement

It is customary to begin with a reintroduction and an explanation, such as: 'I am a doctor who helps children of your age with their problems and muddles' (not a teacher). Children should be told that they will be returned to their parents after a talk. They should be asked why they think they have come.

Children aged at least 6 years

Children will often be on the defensive, knowing that complaints have been made to the doctor about their behaviour. It is, therefore, usually unwise to make any mention of the complaints at the beginning of the interview. The doctor should make it clear by the way they behave towards the children that they are not acting as a judge or as someone who is going to correct or criticize. The aim is rather to show respect for the children as individuals and show interest in what they say and do.

If children are expected to sit down for part of the interview, restless or uninhibited behaviour will be more readily observed. The first aim is to get them relaxed and talking freely, to assess the relationship they are able to form in such a setting, the level and lability of their mood, their conversation, and any habitual mannerisms. In order to provide an adequate sample of behaviour, there should be about 15 minutes of unstructured conversation. The children should be encouraged to talk about recent events and activities, what sort of things they like doing after school and at weekends, what they do with their friends and families, the games they play, what they enjoy and do not enjoy at school, etc. They may also be asked about their hopes for the future, and what they want to do when they leave school or are grown up.

Respond with interest, concern, or enthusiasm, as appropriate (to set a relaxed and informal atmosphere, to try to elicit a range of emotions, and to assess the emotional responsiveness of the child and the kind of relationship they form with the examiner). The interview must be geared to the child's age, intelligence, and interests. If the emotional responsiveness of the child is to be adequately assessed, it is also necessary for the psychiatrist to show a range of emotions (being more serious or concerned when asking about feelings of distress or worry, and more lively when responding to children's accounts of what interests or amuses them).

They should also be asked if they have any friends, what are their names, what they do together, and how they get on with other children at home and at school. Emotionally loaded topics should be pursued as they arise. The examiner's response should not block or lead away from expression of pathology or discomfort.

The children should then be questioned sympathetically about the specific information that should be elicited. Open questions are usually preferable and multiple choice questions are sometimes useful. Specific examples of relevant feelings or events should be asked for. Indirect statements — 'I knew a boy once about your age who …' may be productive. If the child accepts this convention there is no need to challenge it with statements such as, 'this boy is you, isn't he?'

It is expedient to ease off topics that seem too threatening, but the interviewer should return to them. Does the child ever feel lonely, get into fights, get teased, or picked on? Are they picked on more than most other children? Why do they think they are picked on? Similarly, they should be asked how they get on with their brothers and sisters. If they get into fights, do they like fighting, are they 'real' fights or 'friendly' fights?

The children should be asked specifically about worries, ruminations, fears, unhappiness, bad dreams, and the sort of things that make them feel angry. For example, they might be asked: 'Most people tend to worry about some things. What kind of things do you worry about? Do you ever lie awake at night worrying about things? Do you ever get nasty thoughts on your mind that you cannot get rid of? Do you ever get fed up? Miserable? Cry? Feel really unhappy?' Suicidal thoughts should be pursued where appropriate. 'Are there things you are particularly afraid of? What about the dark? Spiders? Dogs? Monsters? Do you ever dream? What about bad dreams? Do you have nightmares? What kind of things make you angry and annoyed?'

If anything positive should come up in answer to these questions, the psychiatrist should probe for the severity, frequency, and setting of the emotions (for instance, 'Do you ever feel so miserable that you want to go away and hide? Or that you want to run away? When was the last time that happened? How often do you feel like that? What sort of things make you fed up? Do you feel like that at home? at school, etc.').

Children can be very suggestible and will sometimes produce answers they think the doctor wants. However, the anxious or depressed child can usually be distinguished by the affective state when talking about worries, fears, feeling fed-up, etc. Although it is important to ask the child systematically about these issues, it is also necessary for much of the interview to consist of neutral or cheerful topics. Note whether the child spontaneously mentions worries or extends answers on those topics beyond the questions.

The child should be asked to draw a picture of someone or a house and everyone who lives in it, and encouraged to talk about it. This provides the opportunity to assess their natural skills, persistence and distractibility, and also their attitudes and feelings, in so far as they are expressed in the drawing and what they say about the drawing. Handedness and fine motor skills can be assessed at the same time.

To assess attention span, persistence and distractibility; children should be given some tasks within their ability, but near to its limits. The drawing constitutes one task; in addition, they might be asked to give days of the week forwards and backwards, the months of the year, and also do some simple arithmetic (such as serial 7s from 100, serial 3s from 30, addition, subtraction, or multiplication tables). This is one situation in the interview where the child is stressed; emotionally loaded discussion is another. Tics and involuntary movements are often at their most apparent when the child is under stress, and should also be noted throughout the interview.

Note that *tics* are rapid, stereotyped, repetitive, non-rhythmic, predictable, purposeless contractions of functionally related muscle groups, which can usually be imitated or suppressed voluntarily for a time; *stereotypies* are voluntary, repeated, isolated, identical, predictable, often rhythmic actions, in which whole areas of the body are involved; *mannerisms* are odd, stylized embellishments of goal-directed movement. Notice also whether the level of activity is increased: *restlessness* is an inability to remain in the seat appropriately; while *fidgetiness* refers to squirming in the seat, or movements of parts of the body, but not the whole child.

Children aged below 6 years

A play-setting will usually be more appropriate for a child of 6 years of age or less: depending on the maturity of the child, it may sometimes be desirable to use a play-interview with older children.

Games and toys should be chosen: (1) to be suitable for the child's age, sex, and social background; (2) to provide an interaction with the interviewer, and (3) to encourage communication and imaginative play. The psychiatrist should get used to using a small range of toys, for example farm animals, colours, a doll's house with figures, plasticine. Board games like chess are not very productive. Imaginative games such as the squiggle game (making a drawing out of the child's squiggle and getting the child to do the same out of your squiggle), playing with family figures, etc., may offer the best opportunity for eliciting a range of behaviour and emotions. Where possible, the child should be seen without the parents. However, with very young children it may often be better to allow the mother to come in with the child first and then, after a short while, she can withdraw from the situation or leave the room.

It is important to allow the child to get used to the situation before the examiner makes an approach. Initially, it may be useful simply to let the child explore the room and the toys while the doctor makes a friendly remark or two, and responds to the child's approaches but making no direct approach. The speed with which the child may be engaged in interaction and the way in which the approach is best made will vary considerably and must be judged in relation to each individual child. An attempt should be made to provide some activity known to interest the child.

The play situation should be utilized to make the same kind of assessment with the older child, and, where appropriate, the child should be questioned in a manner suitable for their level of maturity. Young children cannot be expected to give descriptions of how they feel or to answer complex questions with long words about abstract concepts. Nevertheless, many can explain what they do at home, who they play with, etc.

Sources of information

Children are usually referred as a result of adult concern about the child's behaviour. Much more reliance is placed on accounts derived from a variety of informants than is usual in adult psychiatry. One needs accounts of the child's behaviour and emotions at home, at school or playgroup, and as observed during the assessment.

The child is continually developing. Symptoms and behaviour problems change with developmental stages, as do emotional needs. Even more than with adults, the assessment of behaviour and mental state needs to focus especially on these aspects relevant to the individual child's developmental stage.

Children's social and personal development is strongly influenced by the relationships formed at home and at school. The attitudes of, and the quality of relationships with, adult care-givers need assessment as well as the child's development.

Interviewing parents

The history-taking involves two steps: (1) the obtaining information about events and behaviour; and (2) recording expressed feelings, emotions, or attitudes concerning these events or the individuals participating in them. Because much of the interview is concerned with eliciting precise factual material, it is important to establish early on that the interviewer is interested in feelings as well as events. Care should be taken to encourage positive and negative attitudes to an equal extent. Where the informant's feelings are in doubt, questions such as; 'Does this kind of thing ever cause an atmosphere in the home?', or: 'Does that ever make you feel on edge?' are also useful, but should be used sparingly. In assessing the informant's feelings and emotions attention should be paid to the way things are said as well as to what is said. Differences in the tone of voice — shown in the speed, pitch, and intensity of speech — can be important in the recognition of emotions. Particular attention should be paid to expressed criticism, hostility, and warmth, and to whom it is directed. Facial expressions and gestures should also be taken into account.

It is desirable, when possible, to see both the mother and the father. The child's relationship with their father is as important as that with their mother — although its importance will be for somewhat different aspects of development. It is undesirable to have to rely only on a second-hand account of the father obtained from the mother. An interview with both parents together will often provide a good opportunity for observing parental interaction and relationships. If the parents are divorced or separated and the child spends time with each of them it may be more appropriate to see the other parent on a separate occasion, as well as seeing any new, significant adults in the family.

Present complaint

The interview with the parents begins with an enquiry about the problems or difficulties which are the chief cause of concern to the informant. The parents should tell their story in their own words and then be asked if there are any other difficulties. *Recent examples* of the problems should always be obtained as well as the *frequency* of the behaviour, the *severity*, and the *context* of its occurrence (for example, at school or when the child is away from home). The circumstances which *antecede or precipitate* the behaviour and those which *ameliorate or aggravate* the difficulties should always be noted. Determine the time of onset of the difficulties and go back to the point in the child's development when behaviour or emotions first appeared unusual, abnormal, or a cause for concern. Were there stresses at that time?

This part of the interview gives a good opportunity to assess parental feelings and attitudes, as well as beliefs about the problem; and these should be carefully described. In addition, the interviewer should find out what strategies have been used to deal with the problem, and how much success or failure they have had with each method. It is useful, too, at this point to find out what effect the symptom(s) has had on the rest of the family. If appropriate, the interviewer should also enquire what led to the seeking of help with regard to the child's problem and why help has been sought now rather than at any other time.

If delayed or deviant development is prominent, whether global or specific, turn to p. 38.

Systematic questioning

Typical day

A time budget helps to establish the context for children who are being assessed. In term time, who wakes up first? What happens? Who gets breakfast? How do the children behave first thing? How long do they take to get dressed? Who takes them to school? What are they like when they get home? What do they do then? How closely are they supervised? How do they behave during the evening meal; and when they are going to bed? What are the activities, and who provides care, during the school holidays? (NB This enquiry is essentially to establish the framework; do not spend a long time on meticulous recording of exact details.)

Emotions

Are they happy or miserable? What makes them cry? Are they worried, depressed, suicidal, irritable, sulky? Do they show temper? Exhibit fears and panics? Are there tears on getting to school, or even school refusal? Are they fussy? Are there specific things or situations that arouse fear? Are there any compulsions to do things? (NB Obsessions and compulsions in children are not necessarily accompanied by a subjective sense of resistance and may present as a handicapping ritual that cannot be explained.)

Antisocial trends

Are they disobedient? Destructive? Do they set fires? Tell lies? Steal? Are these problems only at home or outside? Do they happen when alone or with others? How are the problems dealt with? Has there been truanting or running away? Do they smoke, drink, sniff glue, or take drugs? Are they cruel to animals? Has there been any trouble with the police? *If yes to any of these, obtain details and enquire about the child's attitudes to discipline.*

General health

Are they off school at all? Do they suffer from asthma, headaches, stomach aches, or bilious attacks? How good is their sight and hearing?

Eating, sleeping, elimination

Are there eating difficulties at home or at school? Do they show food refusal or faddiness? Pica? Do they have sleeping difficulties — poor settling at night, waking in the night, nightmares? What are the sleeping arrangements? Is there enuresis — diurnal or nocturnal? Wetting when away from home? Have they ever been dry? Is there soiling or smearing? Have they ever been clean? Where is the lavatory? (Regularity of function is also a temperamental attribute.)

Activity and concentration

Are they overactive or restless? Will they stay still if expected to, or are they always fidgety? How good is their concentration and what is the longest time they can concentrate on something interesting? Is there any change or loss of interest?

Motor

Do they have any twitches? Where? Headbanging? Habits or rituals? Do they show clumsiness? Is there preference for a particular hand and foot?

Speech

Do they speak as well as others of the same age, or do they have difficulty in understanding or producing speech, or in pronunciation, such as a lisp, baby talk or stutter? *If marked difficulties, see to Table 2.1.*

Attack disorders

Do they suffer from fainting, fits, or absences? *Obtain details and see section on seizure disorders*

Peer relationships

Although poor peer relationships are not a specific disorder, they are a good indicator of general adjustment.

What are the names of any friends? What do they do together? How close are they, how long have they been friends, do they visit each others' houses? Do other children reject or ignore? Does the child seek social contact or prefer to be solitary? Are peer relationships only with a deviant group?

Relationships with sibs

How do they get on? Is the child particularly attached to any siblings? How is this shown? Are there squabbles and with whom? Do they come to blows? Is there jealousy?

Relationships with adults

(This is also a convenient time to discover parental attitudes.)

How does the child get on with their mother/father? How is affection shown? Are they an easy child to get on with? How do they compare with other children? Whom do they take after and how?

How do they get on with other adults? With teachers? Is there anyone they are particularly attached to? Does anyone help to look after them? What is it about them that parents find hardest to tolerate?

Sex

Is there interest in the opposite sex? Is there development of menarche, body hair, and masturbation? Have they been instructed about sex, asked questions, or had any sexual experience? Is there any inappropriate sexual behaviour?

Present schooling

Which school do they attend? Do they like it? Are their progress reports satisfactory? Has a parent seen the child's teacher? (*See p. 36.*)

Strengths

What are the child's good qualities, abilities, and attractive attributes?

Family history and circumstances

Describe the appearance, manner, and mental state of parental informant(s).

Family structure

Persons in the home: obtain a list. It may be helpful to draw a family tree (see pp. 8–9). Ask about age, religion, occupation, education, and health of each person. Have the child's parents been married before? Are they adopted or fostered? Mother's pregnancies — including miscarriages and stillbirths. Make sure biological parents are identified. Get the same details about a parent or sibs who live away from home.

For important people outside the home — for example, grandparents and parental sibs — establish what contact there is and the child's relationship. Obtain a sketch of the parent's own childhood.

Family history

A history of disorders in biological relatives needs to be taken carefully, because of the importance of genetic factors. For each first-degree relative one should question to determine the presence or absence of any psychiatric disorders, psychiatric treatment, depression, suicide, language delay, difficulty learning to read, enuresis, social oddness, alcoholism, epilepsy, court appearances. Age of onset is helpful. For the more extended family, establish not only which members of the family, if any, have had mental problems but their exact position in the family, and the other members who have not had problems. The pattern of transmission, if there is a familial disorder, needs to be established.

Home circumstances

A home visit is not undertaken routinely, but when indicated it provides the best quality information and can often throw light on puzzling aspects of the history. Does the child live in a house or flat? How many rooms are there? Are there others in the home? What are the sleeping arrangements? Facilities (bath, lavatory, etc.)?

Other care arrangements

Does anyone else look after them — grandparents, childminder, neighbour after school, au pair, divorced parent at weekends, etc.? Have social services been involved? If not living with natural parents, what is the legal status of care?

Finances

What sources of finance are there? Are there any difficulties?

Neighbourhood

How long has the child lived there? Give a description of the area. Is it liked or disliked? Is there conflict with their neighbours? Is there any environmental threat; for instance, frequent assaults?

Family life and relationships

Parental relationships

How do the parents get on with each other? What things do they enjoy doing together? How do they spend evenings and week-ends? To what extent does the father participate in child care, discipline, and household tasks?

Parent–child interaction

What activities are performed by parent and child jointly? Do they go out together? Play together? Help with homework? Help make things?

Child's participation in family activities

Does the child help with dressing, feeding, etc? Who helps? Does the child help with the washing-up, shopping, errands, etc.?

Family pattern of relationships

Are they their mother's child or father's child? Do they confide in their father or in their mother? What attachments to other adults are there?

Rules at home

Do they have bedtime rules? Do they climb on furniture? Leave the house without saying where they're going, etc.? Are there restrictions on friends, staying out late, reading or TV? Who monitors the child's behaviour? Who reprimands? What method of punishment is used? Do they have pocket money?

The child

Personal history

A general account of the art of eliciting a developmental history is to be found on p. 38.

Pregnancy

Was it planned or not, and in what circumstances? (For example, adverse reaction of mother's own parents, abandoned by baby's father.) Were there complications such as toxaemia or haemorrhage; or stresses such as infection, smoking, alcohol, drugs, or X-rays?

Delivery

Enquire about place of birth — home or hospital; length of labour, presentation, mode of delivery, maturity, birthweight, complications? Was resuscitation given — incubator or Special Care Baby Unit? Give details of the mother's health during and after pregnancy including depression.

Neonatal period

Were there difficulties breathing or sucking? Cyanotic attacks? Convulsions? Jaundice? Floppiness? Infection? Were they kept in hospital longer than usual?

Feeding in infancy

Were they breast or bottle fed? When were they weaned? Were there difficulties?

Sleep pattern in infancy

Normal sleep? Describe any difficulties.

Social development in infancy

Were they placid or active? Irritable? What was the child's response to their mother? Did they cry a lot? What other attachments did they have?

Milestones

Useful stages to ask about, include: sitting unsupported, walking unaided, first word with meaning, and first two-word phrases.

Comparison with siblings' development is helpful when exact stages are not remembered.

Bladder and bowel control

When were they dry by day and by night? (This is expected by the age of 5 years.) When did they have bowel control? (This is expected by the age of 4 years.) Were there any difficulties? Was training used? — if so, how was it done? Who trained — child-minders, nurseries, playgroups? — How did they respond?

Allergies

Any evidence of abnormal reactions to drugs or particular foods or drinks?

Illnesses

Were they ever in hospital — in-patient, out-patient, clinic, operations, accidents? Have they had any serious illnesses — measles, meningitis, encephalitis, fits or convulsions?

Separations

Have they ever been away from home without their parents or been separated while in hospital? Have they been apart from their parents for as long as 4 weeks? How were they looked after? What were the circumstances? How did they react?

Failures of care

Has there been any serious adversity in the past? Has caring been inadequate at any point (for example, illness incapacity or absence of a parent)? Has the child ever been maltreated (for instance, by physical or sexual abuse)?

Previous schools

Which schools have they attended? How did they get on? Why were they changed? Has only teacher ever expressed concern to the parents? Has any statement of special needs been made?

Temperamental or personality attributes

It is not easy to disentangle the child's premorbid characteristics from the present problems, but an attempt should be made. Some aspects of temperament are best shown in the response to new situations, new events, and new people, but attention should also be paid to mode of functioning in routine situations.

Meeting new people

What is the child's behaviour with adults? With children? Do they go up to strangers? Are they shy or clinging? How quickly do they adapt to someone new?

New situations

How do they react to new places, new gadgets, and new foods? Do they explore or hang back? How quick are they to adapt?

Emotional expression

How vigorous are they in expressing their feelings? Do they whimper or howl? Chuckle or roar with laughter? How happy/ miserable were they before the present problems? How do they show their feelings?

Affection and relationships

Are they affectionate? Do they confide in anybody, and if so, who? What friendships have they formed?

Sensitivity

How do they respond to a person or animal being hurt? What is their reaction if they have done something wrong?

Information from school and other sources outside the family

Parental consent should always be obtained to contact any agency other than the referrer and the family doctor. In medico-legal work consent is needed to contact any agency other than the referrer. Permission to contact the school and other involved agencies can be requested when the first appointment is sent. If permission is not given for a key contact, such as with the family doctor, then it needs to be sought with a detailed discussion and an explanation of its importance.

A teacher's account of the child's behaviour at school is indispensable.

Ask for information about:

- attendance
- academic strengths and weaknesses
- non-academic skills; for example, art, music, woodwork, sports, etc.
- behaviour in the classroom and playground
- social relationships with teachers and peers
- any other observations of importance.

For preschool children a report along the same lines from a nursery or playgroup leader is of similar importance. It can be helpful to have this information available at the first assessment.

It is good practice to explain to the family that a letter will be sent to the family doctor after the assessment and a request made to obtain old medical records, etc. The family doctor frequently possesses further essential information. In medico-legal work the final report will be sent only to the referrer who will then distribute it to the appropriate parties.

Psychological testing will usually be an important part of the systematic assessment of a child and will usually provide quantified information from behaviour and performance in a rigorously controlled setting. Such an assessment needs to be interpreted in the light of the validity of the test and the nature of the problem. A low test score from an uncooperative child should not necessarily be taken as implying a limitation of intellectual potential. A normal or high IQ score, in a child with problems in everyday learning, does not necessarily entail a non-cognitive explanation: there may be impairment in aspects of cognition that are not assessed by the tests used. If the clinical appraisal of cognitive functioning is discrepant with the psychometric evaluation, then further enquiry is needed to find out why.

Synthesizing different sources

Evidence often conflicts. There is no single rule for how to resolve disagreements; clinical judgement is required.

When there is disagreement, first evaluate whether any of the sources is likely to be unreliable. Is the mother depressed and exaggerating psychopathology; or fearful of the consequences of the assessment and suppressing problems? Have the parents read accounts of disorders such as autism and presented a 'textbook' account? Does a teacher have insufficient acquaintance with the child to be accurate?

Next, consider whether disagreement comes from varying standards about what is expected from a child. Care-givers vary greatly in their beliefs about the degree of deviance required before they decide that a problem is present. It will not be enough to establish that a parent considers, for example, that their child is hyperactive. Rather, detailed enquiry will be needed to establish actual behaviours — such as the length of time the child engages in constructive activities and how long they can remain still in a given situation. Parents are often much better at recalling of behavioural details than at judging what is the range of normality; so apparent disagreements may disappear on close enquiry.

For some problems, priority should be given to one source of information. Children describe their depressed feelings more frequently than adults recognize them. Parental account may, therefore, be insensitive, and the rule is often adopted that the symptom of depression is present if *any* informant gives a clear account of a marked problem in the child. By contrast, antisocial conduct may be denied by the child — especially if parents are present; here the parental account is often more sensitive.

For many problems, accounts may differ because the child is different in different situations. This specificity to context is in itself important diagnostic information: for example hyperactivity that is pervasive across all information sources is more likely to be based on neurodevelopmental dysfunction than the same behaviour seen only in one setting, such as school.

Finally, if doubt persists after careful enquiry and consideration of possible reasons, then the best way of resolving disagreements is for the psychiatrist to make observations directly in the child's natural settings.

The assessment of children with developmental disorders

It is usually most convenient to begin with a chronological account of the child's development. Records of previous developmental assessments should be requested, but parental account is still needed. However, rather than go immediately to questions of the pregnancy and delivery, it may be preferable to start by asking the parents when they first became concerned that something might be not quite right with their child's development, and what it was that aroused their concern at the time. Particularly with a first child, the parents' concern may have been aroused long after the child first showed delays or distortions in development. It is helpful to enquire whether, with hindsight, the parents think that all was well before they first became concerned and, if not, what it was that might have been abnormal. Having established the time and nature of those first indications of concern, it is generally easiest to go back to the time of pregnancy and work forward systematically up to the present time. Most parents do not accurately remember when milestones were reached if they were within the normal range, but they are more likely to recall them if they were delayed. It is helpful to focus on that aspect first before going on to tie down the time more exactly. When seeking to date milestones reference should be made to familiar landmarks rather than to ages as such. It might be appropriate, for example, to ask whether the child was walking on his first birthday, or when they moved house, or at the time of his first Christmas, or when the second child was born.

Particular attention needs to be paid to the developmental aspects of play, socialization, and language. With respect to the milestones of language it is crucial to be quite specific about what is being asked. Parents are very inclined to interpret all manner of sounds as speech, and especially as 'mama' and 'dada'. Consequently, it may be wise to ask very focused questions such as: 'When did he first use simple words with meaning — that is words other than mama and dada?' 'What were his first words?'; and, 'How did he show that he knew their meaning?'. In addition to the first use of single words it is important to ask about babble, the use of two- or three-word phrases, the use of pointing, gesture, or mime, the following of instructions, and immediate or delayed echoing. It is helpful to identify some occasions that the parents remember reasonably clearly and then to focus on what the child was like at that time. In doing so, an attempt should be made to determine what the child was like at about 2 years, 30 months, 3 years, and 4 years.

Few parents think of socialization in terms of milestones or indeed in terms of specific behaviours. As a result, although the topic may be introduced by some general question such as: 'How affectionate was he as a toddler?', it will always be necessary to proceed with a series of focused questions directed at eliciting information in key aspects of social relationships and social responsiveness at particular ages. Thus, for the 6–12-month age period it would be necessary to ask whether the child turned to look the parents directly in the face when they spoke to him, whether he put up his arms to be lifted, whether he nestled close when held, whether he protested when left, whether he laughed and chortled in response to parental overtures, whether he was comforted by being picked up and cuddled, and whether he was wary of strangers. Similarly with toddlers, questions should be asked about whether the child greeted a parent coming home, whether he sought to be cuddled when upset or hurt ('did he come to you or did you have to go to him?'); whether he differentiated between parents and others in whom he went to for comfort; whether he showed separation anxiety; and whether he could be playful, and enter into the spirit of to and fro in a teasing or make-believe game.

The psychiatric interview with children **39**

Precise questions are required to elicit an adequate account of the child's play at particular ages. Thus, to determine whether play was normal at 2 years of age the clinician should ask about the child's use of toys and other objects. Did he or she recognize the appropriate use of miniature toys — by pushing toy cars along the floor and making car noises, or rather did they tend to spin the wheels, feel the texture of the paint, or listen to the sound of a wind-up car? Was there any pretend play — as with the use of toy tea-sets, dolls, etc?. Would the pretend play vary from day to day and would the pretend element be used to create any sort of sequence of story (with the toy cars racing each other, being parked in the garage, or being used to go to Granny's home)?

Having obtained a history of the development of play, social interaction, and language — with special reference to the first 5 years — it is necessary to obtain a comparably specific account of the child's *current behaviour* in these areas of functioning. Before proceeding to direct questioning on particular features it is helpful to get an overall picture of the child's activities by asking how he spends his time on returning from school or at a weekend. Such a description usually provides a lifelike portrayal of the bleakness or richness of the child's inner and outer world, and focuses attention on the activities and experiences to be asked about in greater detail. For adequate evaluation to be possible, the specific questioning should be based on a systematic scheme that ensures that each of the crucial areas is covered, as set out in Tables 2.1–3.

Table 2.1 Scheme for current speech and language

1. *Imitation* — of housework, etc.
2. *Inner language* — meaningful use of miniature objects, pretend play, drawing
3. *Comprehension of gesture*
4. *Comprehension of spoken language*

   Hearing: response to sounds; response to being called by name; reaction to loud noises; reaction to quiet, meaningful sounds (mother's footsteps, noise of a spoon in a dish, food being prepared, door opening, rattle, etc.); ever thought deaf?

   Listening and attention

   Understanding: response to simple and complicated instructions with and without gesture (get details of examples)
5. *Vocalization and babble (non-speaking child)*

   Amount

   Complexity

   Quality

   Social usage — does he babble back to you?
6. *Language production*

   Mode: gesture, pointing; taking by hand; speech

   Complexity: syntactical and semantic; length of sentences; vocabulary; use of personal pronouns, etc.

   Qualities: echoing, stereotyped features, I–you confusion, made-up words, other oddities

   Amount

   Use of social communication: asking for things; to comment or chat to and fro; in reply to questions; mute in certain situations
7. *Word-sound production*

   Any difficulties in pronunciation: consonants omitted or substituted; which ones; slurring; dysarthria; nasality. Are speech defects consistent or variable?
8. *Phonation* and volume of speech
9. *Prosody*: pattern of stress and tonal variation in speech
10. *Rhythm*: abnormalities of rhythm: stuttering, lack of cadence and inflection; coordination with breathing.

Table 2.2 Scheme for current social interaction

1. *Differentiation between people* — shown by different responses to mother, father, stranger, etc.

2. *Selective attachment*
   Source of security or comfort, to whom does he go when hurt?
   Greeting — for example, parent returning from work
   Separation anxiety

3. *Social overtures*
   Frequency and circumstances; appropriateness to the situation
   Quality: visual gaze, facial expression, and enthusiasm

4. *Social responses*
   Frequency and circumstances
   Quality: eye-to-eye gaze, facial expression, and emotions
   Reciprocity: to and fro dialogue

5. *Social play*
   Playfulness
   Spontaneous imitation
   Cooperation and reciprocity, sharing
   Emotional expression
   Pleasure in the other person
   Humour
   Social excitement

Table 2.3 Scheme for current play.

1. *Social aspects* (see Table 2.2)

2. *Cognitive level*
   Curiosity
   Understanding how things work
   Complexity: puzzles, drawing, rule-following, inventiveness
   Imagination: pretend play, creativity, spontaneity, telling stories

3. *Content, type, and quality*
   Initiation
   Variable or stereotyped
   Unusual preoccupations
   Unusual object attachments
   Rituals and routines
   Resistance to change
   Stereotyped movements
   Interest in unusual aspects of people or objects

4. *Attention*
   Orientation to a new situation and a new toy
   Distractibility to extraneous stimuli
   Length of time playing with each toy, and frequency of change of activity
   Persistence vs. leaving play activities unfinished
   Acceptance of, and persistence with, toys or activities introduced by the examiner

3
Special assessments with adults

Family relationships

There are many reasons why it can be valuable to interview the family of the presenting patient (index patient), ranging from obtaining a good description of fits, and other altered states of consciousness to an examination of the family dynamics, for example to uncover possible maintaining influences in relation to the patient who relapses when a discharge date is decided. The index patient is, of course, included in the family meeting.

As a general rule, the earlier the family can be included in the investigation and treatment of a problem, the better, assuming the index patient is agreeable. It is important for the interviewer to be alert to the strengths and resources of the family who will usually have tried hard to support and help their ill member before calling in the professionals. By the time they see you they may be feeling demoralized and helpless. They may be angry with the patient and secretly blaming themselves or each other. Under these circumstances it is crucial that you do not add to their guilt or sense of failure.

How to manage a family interview

After initial introductions and an explanation of the setting — one-way screen, closed-circuit TV, etc. — start by thanking the family members for coming and acknowledging interruptions to school and work. Then state the purpose of the meeting by inviting them to assist you in helping the index patient — as indeed they are experts by virtue of having known him for longer and before he became ill. It is usually best to start by asking for a description of the problem, being sure to hear the views of each member of the family for their perception of the problem.

Even at this early stage one often gets startlingly different descriptions of the problem. It is valuable to define the problem as it affects the family now and to clarify that this may be different from how the problem began. The focus at this early stage in the interview is to translate the problem (described as an attribute of the index patient) into statements about relationships and differences in relationships among the family members. At all times it is important to note their non-verbal messages: posture, eye contact, interruptions, and emotional states; detachment, fear, sadness, etc.

One may enquire into current alliances in relation to the present problem — who feels most upset (by the problem), who notices first, who gets impatient first — obtaining a ranking of all members in relation to each question. It is very useful to track sequences of behaviour around the problem as this provides a detailed pattern of activity which is often stereotypic.

It is the family's attempt at a solution which has itself become part of the problem. By asking different family members for their explanation of how the pattern has evolved or why particular members take up particular roles in the sequence of behaviour it is usually possible to uncover differences of opinion about what happens. It can be useful to ask what other approaches to the problem have been tried and why they were abandoned.

When you feel you have a clear picture of how the family tries and fails to help in relation to the immediate problem it is time to enquire into how the problem affects other aspects of the family's life together. How does the family regroup when the index patient is ill, or away in hospital? Who takes over their tasks, who misses them most? By comparing current arrangements and role assignments with those before the problem began, certain hypotheses about what function the problem serves will emerge.

The final part of an initial family interview involves establishing with the family members whether or not they are willing to continue to work together with you in arriving at a better understanding of the problem and finding a way either of resolving it or living with it. Alternatively, you may discover there is such hostility towards the index patient or so much chaos, discord, or obstructiveness that it is clear the patient will have to be helped to live apart from his family. Although painful — this is usually much better accepted by the patient if the limits of what each family member is willing to offer in terms of help and support is clear to him. For example, a couple who have both divorced and remarried each had to say to their adult, chronic schizophrenic daughter, in front of each other 'You cannot, under any circumstances, live with me'. In this case, the previous uncertainty had been perpetuated by each one saying 'Wait until you are better, then you can live with me or possibly the other parent'.

There is so much information to take in, record, and interpret in a family interview that it is of great value to have an non-involved observer or a video recording. Any kind of electronic record requires the informed consent of the family, at the beginning of the interview, with the option to delete the recording at the end.

Your observations may be recorded under the following headings:

Description of family members present

The family includes all those currently living in the same household; but children who have left home and relatives in other households who are significantly involved may also be included.

- Note absent members.
- List names, ages, physical appearance, and mental state.

Description of the problem

- Use the words of the family members.
- Include the problem as it began and the problem now.
- Record any stereotypic pattern if elicited.

The stage of family life cycle

- Courtship, marriage, and the honeymoon period.
- The first child alters the couple's view of themselves and each other as they make space for the baby.
- Subsequent children each make demands for adjustment on existing family members.
- The children reach adolescence: the onset of puberty and sexual awakenings, bids for independence with the challenge of leaving home.

- The 'empty nest' as the last child leaves home. The couple, having reached midlife or later, face the dependence, illness, or death of their own parents, as well as what remains of their own life together. Crises in families often arise when transition to the next stage is required, but which, for some reason, cannot be successfully negotiated. Crises may result in a symptomatic member or marital difficulties may occur, or both.

The genogram or family tree

This can be a powerful tool for eliciting transgenerational resonances. It is important to ask about stillbirths and other premature deaths; note the ages and the date of death of grandparents, siblings, and children. Crises in the life cycles of the previous generation (the parents families of origin) may illuminate difficulties in the presenting family. The occupations of each person should be indicated, if known, (see also pp. 8–9).

The family structure

This refers to the existence of appropriate or inappropriate boundaries between different parts of the family: the boundary between the couple and each of their families of origin, as well as parents and children. Are there transgenerational alliances — father and daughter; mother and son; grandmother, mother, and daughter? Is one member of the family isolated (for example, the father) or scapegoated (for example, a child who is different from the other siblings)? Facts informing these judgements can be elicited by asking about the routine daily activities. Who does what with whom? How are mealtimes, bed times, housework, household chores, and leisure activities arranged? How are decisions made — do the couple consult one another? If not, who gets consulted and who does not? How are conflicts negotiated and resolved? Who has the final say? Who controls the finances? In families with an ill adolescent, the hierarchy is sometimes inverted, the parents are capriciously governed by their offspring.

Family roles and attitudes

In response to the questions above it should also become clear whether particular family members are assigned, by common agreement, to certain roles; and how power, authority, and gender-specific activities are distributed. Implicit in these roles will be shared attitudes; although when made explicit, differences of opinion may emerge. Acceptance of role-assignment may be a way of avoiding conflict. Cultural and religious attitudes are often expressed in role assignments and expectations based on gender and birth order. A good way to find out more about cultural and religious views with which the interviewer is unfamiliar is to acknowledge difference and ignorance and ask. It also allows the family members to describe what it is like for them to belong to an ethnic minority and the impact the dominant culture makes on their lives.

Communication and emotional climate

These aspects of the description of family relationships will first of all depend upon your observations of the family when they respond to your questioning. Supplementary questioning can clarify how the various family members experience and think about each other. If, for example, the mother tends to answer for her daughter, one can ask the daughter: 'Does your mother always know what you are thinking?', or ask the father or other relative: 'how does your daughter manage to get her mother to speak for her?', or ask a sibling 'Does your mother always speak for your sister or are there times when your sister can speak for herself?'.

Other common patterns are: one family member is frequently interrupted by another, one member is habitually silent and ignored, or disengaged, or over-emotional; everyone talks at once; no one finishes a sentence; no one listens to anyone else; one member habitually defers to another.

There may be obvious omissions or evasions. Communication may be clear and direct or contradictory or obfuscating.

The emotional atmosphere may be free or frozen, cool and distant, or intensely over-involved. Dyads or subsystems may be locked in superiority and submission, condescension and self-effacement, cruelty and humiliation.

The hypothesis

This is an attempt to describe the problem in systemic terms, that is what maintains and prevents resolution of the problem in terms of the contribution each family member who, it is predicted, both gains and suffers from the status quo.

Assessment of early life experience

High-risk patients — most will be mentally ill

In the absence of a suitable informant, the patient may only be able to report what they have been told about their early years, the period of normal childhood amnesia. If they report amnesia for most of their childhood there must be a strong suspicion that there have been events too painful to remember which have been actively obliterated. Significant events which probably will have influenced the person's early development, coping strategies, personality, relationship patterns, and vulnerabilities are as follows:

- Puerperal illness of the mother, which led to actual separation or subtle deficiencies in early maternal care.

- Siblings born in rapid succession: pregnancy can interfere with the mother's ability to be receptive to her infant's hostility towards its unborn sibling. This can lead to suppression of feelings of rivalry and jealousy in the child, mistakenly reported as lack of jealousy.

- Twinship stresses the mother, twins, and all the family. Rivalry between twins and their separate development may be obliterated in many ways if the parents find it too painful and complex to deal with. Its reported absence is abnormal.

- Death of a parent and bereavement reactions of the survivors can have a lasting effect. Who helped the subject to mourn?

- Chronic illness, especially mental illness of a parent. Was it a family secret? What help did the family have from outside? Who became the 'parental child'?

- Parental strife and separation inevitably leads to divided loyalties. A mother who cannot separate from a violent partner exposes her children to confusion. They want to but cannot protect her and they cannot understand why she does not leave to protect herself.

- Single parenthood: perhaps poverty, lack of emotional support, frequent changes of sexual partner with an increased risk of child abuse by partners.

- Frequent changes of domicile — ruptures peer relationships and disrupts schooling.

- Bullying at school suggests poor self-esteem, poor social skills, and insecure early attachment pattern.

- Frequent hospitalizations: separations, painful operations, disruption of schooling and peer relations, overanxious or disengaged parents.

- Major environmental failure: in and out of care, foster homes, children's homes, childhood sexual and physical abuse, neglect, emotional deprivation.

Psychiatrists and memories of sexual abuse

Normal memory

To a degree all memories are unreliable. They are not held like video tapes in the mind to be replayed at recall. Rather, when a memory is cued it is processed even prior to the stage when it reaches awareness. This processing can include the incorporation of general knowledge or material from another record. Following the remembering, information will be stored as a record of the remembering. The next time the cycle of remembering is entered the recall may be for the original or may be for the previous recall. Not every detail of an event is stored in memory. When an event is recalled it might need elaborating before it is intelligible to consciousness. What we are conscious of is a mixture of reproduction and reconstruction. Reconstructive memory is characterized by conflation of different events, filling out of detail, and importation of information.

The factors which influence the degree of reconstruction include:

- the personal significance of the event
- its emotive content

- the time elapsed between the event occurring and its recall
- the age at which the event occurred
- the reasons why the person is remembering the event and the circumstances of recall.

Summary of British Psychological Society report

- Highly significant events which evoke deep beliefs, attitudes, and emotional reactions may lead to a narrowing of attention. As a consequence, the peripheral details may be subject to reconstructive error. Repeated events lead to a schematic, generalized representation which can be used as a framework. Individual events become confused. Thus, normal memory is largely accurate but may contain distortions and elaborations.

- With certain exceptions, such as where there has been extensive rehearsal of an imagined event, the source of our memories is generally perceived accurately.

- Nothing can be recalled accurately from before the first birthday and little from before the second. Poor memory from before the fourth birthday is normal.

- Forgetting certain kinds of trauma is often reported, although the nature of the mechanism or mechanisms involved remains unclear.

Absent memories: amnesia for abuse

Children who presented for medical care following sexual abuse were seen as adults, on average 17 years later. Over a third (38 per cent) appeared to have no memory of their early abuse. Loss of memory was most common if the abuse occurred when they were young and was perpetrated by someone they knew.

Recovered false memories

'Recovered memories' usually occur in the context of amnesia at the start of therapy such that clients giving their life history would be unaware of abuse as a child. The memories are reported in the course of therapy which typically employs memory recovery techniques. These include hypnosis (especially hypnotic regression), journalling, guided imagery, guided meditation, and the use of so-called truth drugs.

False beliefs/ inaccurate memories

There is a great deal of evidence for incorrect memories, that is to say where an event has happened but the details are wrongly recalled. This is because of the mental processing, some of it unconscious, that occurs when memories are recollected. The extent to which this occurs is outside the individual's awareness. There is an unstable relationship between confidence and accuracy.

Psychiatric practice and memories of sexual abuse

Obtaining a psychiatric history which may include sexual abuse poses difficulties.

Inaccuracies in psychiatric history

Repeated admissions to psychiatric hospitals leads to the history being recounted on many occasions. What we know about memory is that if there is extensive rehearsal of an imagined event the person can believe the event happened. The memory can become highly detailed and vivid to the person. The event can be altered in matters of detail by suggestion and leading questions. It is common practice for the patient's account to be recorded in psychiatric notes without any attempt to question the source or reliability of the memory. Indeed the American Psychiatric Association report stated:

...psychiatrists should maintain an empathic, non judgmental, neutral stance towards memories of sexual abuse. As in the treatment of all patients, care must be taken to avoid prejudging the cause of the patient's difficulties or the veracity of the patient's reports. A strong belief by the psychiatrist that sexual abuse, or other factors, are or are not the cause of the patient's problems is likely to interfere with appropriate assessment and treatment. Many individuals who have experienced sexual abuse have a history of not being believed by their parents, or others in whom they have put their trust. Expression of disbelief is likely to cause the patient further pain and decrease his/her willingness to seek psychiatric treatment. Similarly clinicians should not exert pressure on patients to believe in events that may have not occurred, or to prematurely disrupt important relationships or make other important decisions based on these speculations....

One of the strongest criteria in assessing the reliability of a memory is the accuracy with which it is anchored in place and time. However, it may be difficult to establish these sort of facts in the context of the approach (empathic non-judgemental) defined above. Thus, the history from the patient may be unreliable and the process of medical treatment may further contribute to faulty recollection.

The mental state and inaccuracies of memory

Abnormal mental states are likely to lead to errors in the reconstruction of memories. This is obvious in psychotic states, but it also occurs in extreme emotional states. In such states of mind there are errors and biases in memory processing and evaluative judgements and in overall information processing.

Informants

The fact that memories can be unreliable is recognized in psychiatry and is why informants are often used to corroborate the history. This is recognized as good psychiatric practice. The history should be compiled from information elicited both from the patient and from one or more informants. The informant's account will not only amplify the patient's report of factual detail but will supplement the patient's account. Clinicians bear a heavy responsibility to do no harm. The desire to help heal the victims of childhood abuse is more than justified, but clinicians are urged to reflect upon the damage done by false accusations. Accepting the truth of long-forgotten memories elicited by therapy without corroboration can seriously injure and disrupt the lives of innocent people.

However, many psychiatrists feel uncomfortable if they attempt to obtain corroboration in this area. They are uncertain what questions they should ask and of whom? Are they not breaking confidentiality if they attempt to do this?

The corroborative evidence useful in a psychiatric history is different from that required for forensic reasons. Open, broad questions can be used. For example, if there is a history of child sexual abuse it would be reasonable to ask the parents, other relatives, and schools whether any difficulties or concerns were noted during the child's development.

Sexual disorders and couple relationship problems

Sexual history

Ask about:

- age at puberty (voice breaking, shaving, menarche)
- age at which first ejaculation occurred
- age at first masturbation — how this was regarded? — fantasies — anxieties
- attitudes of parents to sexual matters
- sexual seduction or childhood sexual abuse
- any unusual sexual preferences — fantasies — activities
- homosexual or heterosexual orientation (fantasies, desires, and experiences)
- any gender dysphoria, including non-arousing cross-dressing
- previous sexual experiences and relationships, including painful or traumatic ones
- current sex life (if any) — marital, extramarital, visiting, or cohabiting
- current frequency of masturbation

- level of sexual drive — any changes during this illness
- contraception, safe sex, sexually transmitted diseases
- sexual dysfunctions — desire, arousal, or orgasm — partner satisfied
- discrepancy in sexual interest between partners
- menopause, hysterectomy, hormone replacement.

Marital and relationship history

Ask about:

- age at first intercourse
- number of previous engagements or serious relationships
- difficulties in these and reasons for break-up
- age at present marriage (or cohabitation) — reasons (e.g. pregnancy)
- age, occupation, health, and personality of partner
- quality of relationship — threat of separation or divorce
- reaction of partner to patient's present illness
- communication, negotiation of differences, ability to confide, empathy
- dominance, submission, distance, trust, fidelity, jealousy
- problems, past and present, arguments, violence
- death of spouse, separation (temporary or permanent), or divorce
- changes in sexual activities during relationship (e.g. ageing effects)
- obstetric history — pregnancies, live births, terminations, and miscarriages.

Children (present or earlier relationships) establish

(1) ages, gender, names, present and past health, any psychiatric problems or treatment; (2) attitude towards children and future

pregnancies; (3) proximity and contact with children not no longer living at home.

Assessment of personality

Definition

Personality is a summary term used to describe traits, attitudes, and behaviours to enable an individual to be identified. Personality, in contrast to symptom states, is largely constant throughout life. Certain personalities are recognized in current psychiatric classifications (ICD-10, DSMIV) which, if accompanied by evidence of suffering for the individual or social handicap, may be diagnosed as personality disorder.

Why assess personality?

Some 10 per cent of psychiatric hospital admissions are patients with a primary diagnosis of personality disorder; around 30 per cent of admissions have personality disorder as an ancillary diagnosis. For yet other patients, the term 'abnormal premorbid personality' is used — where the ICD-10 or DSMIV description of personality is appropriate, but without evidence of distress or handicap.

Who should provide information?

Self-description is difficult and, in a clinical situation, current mental state (for instance, depression, psychosis) may distort the perspective. An informant, someone who has known the patient when they were free of symptoms for a number of years and preferably in more than one circumstance, is desirable. For some personality types, (for example avoidant, anankastic) (obsessional), self-report may be regarded as accurate. The interviewing doctor or ward staff rarely know a patient long enough and in 'normal' circumstances to be sure of personality type. (NB It is important to avoid using the term 'personality disorder' to explain disagreeable behaviour during admission unless you have adequate evidence.)

How should information be classified?

ICD-10 and DSMIV provide categorical typographies of personality disorder: features are listed for each category and the threshold (number of features to be present), with evidence of handicap or suffering to meet the criteria for personality disorder. The clinical assessment, therefore, should aim to discover if one of these categories is appropriate.

A second concept of personality abnormality relevant in psychiatric practice is immaturity. Some individuals will not meet the abnormality above, but show repeated failure accompanied by self-concern and distress to meet key aspects of the adult role — separation from parents, a stable social life or occupation, and a one-to-one relationship. These may indicate difficulty in personality maturation. NB Some individuals who *choose* not to attain any of these aims are excluded from this category.

These two approaches do not classify all humankind. Both the above concepts assess what might be regarded as undesirable features. The informant interview may also yield other aspects of personality, indeed, positive features which should be recorded even when they cannot be classified as a diagnosis.

How should the interview proceed?

It is important to be sure that the informant or patient (as his or her own informant) understands that this interview concerns a time of life when the patient was well. Agree that time with the informant, for example, five years ago or before the marriage broke down, and focus the interview on that period. Begin by asking the informant an open-ended question to describe, in their own words, how the patient was at that time. This response itself may indicate which diagnostic category of personality may be appropriate. However, if uninformative, the following more specific questions will probe for one of the ICD-10 categories:

- How does he/she get on with people? *(paranoid)*
- Does he/she have many friends? *(schizoid)*
- Does he/she trust other people? *(impulsive, paranoid)*
- What is his/her temper like? *(dissocial)*
- How does he/she cope with life? *(anxious, borderline)*
- Is he/she anxious or shy? *(avoidant)*
- How much does he/she depend on others? *(dependent)*
- How does he/she respond to criticism? *(anxious, paranoid)*
- Is he/she over-emotional or irresponsible? *(histrionic, dissocial, borderline)*
- Does he/she have unusually high standards at work or home? *(anankastic)*

Any one of these probes may point to one of the ICD-10 categories. The interviewer should, therefore, follow with subsidiary questions that concern the additional feature of that category (see Appendix 8 for details). In addition, the informant should be asked to indicate whether these features were generally present (for example, not just at work) and whether the personality seemed responsible for personal suffering (for instance, periods of distress or unhappiness) or handicap in social or occupational life. From this information, abnormal premorbid personality may be identified or personality disorder diagnosed.

If the patient is to be the informant, then the same procedure can be followed. It is important under these circumstances to know that it is difficult to be sure that an explosive, impulsive, or antisocial personality is present.

The social state

The social state provides a structure of five main headings, for each of which four main categories of information and assessment can be reported. In practice, the information may be written in columnar form or sequentially down the page. Not all four categories or columns will be needed if significant problems are absent. The format must allow for the possibility that only a very brief or highly distilled report will be required (or feasible) in some cases, while others may require a lot of detailed information. The social state refers to their normal home setting (even if it is a doorway in the street) rather than the place in which the patient is examined. For a long-stay hospital patient, the usual home environment will initially be the ward. The five main headings are: accomodation; finances; home activities; outside activities; carers.

Accommodation

Under this heading are described the physical nature of the patient's residence and the identity of the people who normally provide the immediate social environment. The aim is to assess the type and quality of physical resources available to the patient in the home and to name the people who share the accommodation. Subheadings include:

- type of accommodation
- physical amenities, personal space
- quality of accommodation
- identity of other people sharing the accommodation
- ease of access
- physical security
- nature and quality of neighbourhood.

Finances

This requires a description of the patient's financial status and use of welfare benefits, in order to assess income, monetary assets, liabilities, and capacities to handle money. Subheadings include:

- sources of income (including welfare benefits)
- capital
- expenditure (including special liabilities such as gambling)
- debts (including threats of punitive action such as withdrawal of services or eviction)
- budgeting capacity.

Home activities

The focus here is on daily events and activities within the home, and the provision of both informal and professional support and services from people visiting the home. Subheadings include:

- way of spending a typical day (includes waking and rising, daily routines)
- daily living skills (including personal hygiene, laundry, cooking, cleaning)
- recreational activities
- visitors
- relationships with immediate neighbours.

Outside activities

The patient is seen in relationship to the local and wider community outside the home residence. Subheadings include:

- occupation
- social contacts (family, friends, others)
- shopping
- travel
- use of public amenities (e.g. pubs, cinema)
- other outside leisure activities
- religious observance
- holidays.

Carers

Under this heading are listed the people who are individually identifiable as accepting a special responsibility for promoting and sustaining the patient's welfare. They may include family members, friends, other informal contacts, and members of professional agencies. Subheadings include:

Informal carers

- caring relatives and friends
- relationships with other people within the home and local community

- attitudes to patient reported by others (or observed by assessor) within home;

Professional carers

- staff members of NHS agencies (GP, psychiatric services, etc. — and relationships with them)
- staff members of other statutory agencies (social services, etc.)
- members of voluntary bodies (including religious organizations, etc.).

Each of the above headings is to be recorded using four vertical columns:

Facts — Problems — Services — Strengths

Facts — aims to record the situation in terms of reported objective information from the patient or identified others (including the assessor).

Problems — comprises two elements, which may be reported separately: subjective difficulties reported by the patient and objective difficulties observed by others.

Services — reports provisions already made at the time of assessment to alleviate some, but not necessarily all, of the problems identified. Inadequacies or overprovision may be commented on, but this area of the assessment report is not the place to record proposals about management.

Strengths — invites the assessor to report on positive features of the patient's social opportunities and functioning, which may serve to counterbalance the commonly prevailing negative tone of many psychiatric assessments by highlighting positive resources, relationships and potentialities.

The social state should be recorded *after* the history but *before* the mental state examination. In this position it supplants and extends the information which may at present be recorded in the history, partly under previous personality and partly under social history or current circumstances.

Cross-cultural assessments in psychiatry

The three attributes of awareness, knowledge, and skill could be considered a sequence to be adopted in cross-cultural training. The aim of such a training is to provide the mental health professionals with an insight which encourages you to examine the assumptions that contribute to your behaviour and attitudes when dealing with patients from other cultures. The main goal of this section is to highlight some of the areas which may influence your perception and stereotypes of individuals whose ethnic and racial background and cultural influences may be different from your own. The doctor–patient interaction is affected by the training, past experience, social class, and ethnicity on the doctor's part and by past experiences, educational and social background, and ethnicity of the patient. It is of course likely, that gender, socio-economic or educational status, lifestyle, job, or professional role may overshadow the ethnic or racial identity of the patient.

If the cultural variables are over-emphasized, the provider is guilty of stereotyping the patient, while if these are under-emphasized, the doctor is guilty of insensitivity to the dynamic ranges of influences that may impinge on the interview. Mental health services are frequently looked down upon by members of ethnic minorities because the institutions may be seen to replace support systems, may reflect Western dominant cultural values, may rely on psychological formulations which ignore cultural values and norms of ethnic minorities, and these institutions may be seen to be pandering to those who conform to the dominant culture.

Limitations of psychiatric assessments

These limitations are linked with perceptions that suggest that all people's presentations to psychiatric services can be conceptualized, and their distress fully understood, by mechanistic application of a standardized assessment interview. Duration, content, and focus of psychiatric assessment will depend very much upon the purpose of the assessment whether it is for diagnosis, management, rehabilitation, or psychotherapy. One of the commonest errors in cross-cultural assessments is to foreclose further or detailed enquiry as soon as the psychiatrist believes to have reached a clinical diagnosis.

It is better to use assessment interviews as the basis for beginning to understand a patient's distress and go on to develop a collaborative therapeutic relationship. The common reductionist approach emerges partly because of time restrictions, Western style psychiatric training, necessity to act in an emergency, and recognition that the communication is poor because of linguistic difficulties, but with an uncertainty about the idioms of distress without having had enough time to carry out a more thorough assessment. Some patients, irrespective of their ethnic status, will require a longer assessment before a comprehensive management plan can be formulated so that it truly reflects the *optimal* package of interventions for that particular patient.

The inherent potential inadequacy of psychiatric assessment is amplified where the patient and the clinician come from different cultural backgrounds and for whom the only common reference point is the culture of the clinic.

Box 3.1 Special features of optimal cross-cultural psychiatric assessments

---

- Patients' and their families' expectations of the consultation, and explanations of causes, prognosis and treatment.

- Cultural and religious patterns of communication, taboos, physical distance, religious and other rites of passage.

- Potential for misinterpretation from both sides of consultation especially racism, stereotyping, direct questioning, physical touch, distance, eye contact, linguistic barriers.

- Appraisal properly contextualized in accord with the patient's culture by the involvement of those properly familiar with the patient's culture and preferably with a knowledge of psychiatric nosology.

- Critical appraisal of the limitations the assessment especially where there is a great deal that is unknown.

Communication and cultural distance

The principles outlined here are not a recipe of how to do it culture by culture but are general guidelines aimed at ensuring safe and sensitive practice. It is clearly an advantage if you have some prior understanding of the culture from which your patient comes, and understand something of its essential features, including taboos, rites of passage, and religious values. The first and preferred language in which the patient communicates must be identified prior to commencing the interview. If this is not English, an appropriate interpreter must be identified who can also act as an advisor on non-verbal communication as well as identifying idioms of distress and 'emotional' words used by the patient.

The first step therefore must be an unstructured ten minutes of 'emotional orientation', during which idioms of distress and emotional words can be identified which will give a clue towards the direction in which the assessment must proceed (see Box 3.2).

Box 3.2 Setting up the assessment: use of interpreter

- Be aware of your own culture, and know your limits. Understand that your skills can be blunted by the values of your own culture.

- For each party involved in consultation elicit first language, religion, self-defined ethnicity, identification with specific cultural groups.

- Know the interpreter's role, skills, and limits. Meet with them before the assessment commences to identify their knowledge of culture, identify sources of difference, such as dialect, tribe, religion, island.

- Do not ask children to interpret. Avoid relatives interpreting unless an emergency and delay will be detrimental to the patient.

- Agree on method of joint working — literal translation — cultural context of complaints, any objections to that particular interpreter.

- Emphasize confidentiality to the patient and interpreter.

Essential historical data

Adverse events

Do not assume that the life events, adverse or otherwise, have the same significance for patients as they do for you or that they have only the significance described previously in the literature. Flexible enquiry will accurately elicit the impact of a patient's experiences. Similarly, admission or separation from children may be more traumatic than you might imagine, with culturally unacceptable implications.

World view

This is the patient's perspective of the consultation and the emotional distress leading onto this interaction. It has been described as the personal lens through which people differentially interpret events. This can be further divided into group and individual identity and the patient's beliefs, values, and cognitive perceptions of the distress and the help being offered. This can only be ascertained after several semi-structured meetings with patients, family, advocates, and religious and community spokespersons as nominated by the patient. This will give a profile of events, thought, and approaches to the problems of living deployed by the patient living in a majority culture which may be perceived as hostile. Such a collation of information will provide a culturally contextualized, culturally sensitive information.

Acculturation

No culture remains static. Increasing contact with other cultures by living in close proximity to them along with globalization of cultures, and cultural expectation and behaviour will vary across generations. Acculturation must be seen as a multi-dimensional phenomenon which reflects the changes an individual goes through when he/she is exposed to a new culture. The concept of self varies across cultures, and changes brought about by cultures in individual self will vary across cultures. Acculturation is a feature for the individual, families, religious groups, and other culturally similar local groupings. It is not identical at each level and it is possible that degrees of acculturation will vary across different members of the family. Idioms of distress and expression of such distress, along with help-seeking, are all linked with processes of acculturation. Assess acculturation by determining the period since migration and reasons for migration and by focusing on areas of religious activity, preferred dietary patterns, preferred leisure activities, and attitudes to traditional patterns of behaviour in the community (see Box 3.3).

Box 3.3 Assessment of Acculturation — broad headings

● **Religion**	Practice, identity, frequency of prayer. Who attends? Where? Needs during admission.
● **Languages**	Which languages spoken, degree of literacy. Frequency of use? Which language used for more emotional expression?
● **Marriage/family**	Type-romantic love, degree of autonomy in decision to be married. Attitudes to marriage, children. Responsibility at home? Gender roles?
● **Employment**	Working with others of same ethnicity? Relationships with work colleagues?
● **Leisure activities**	Which interests? Films? Music? Degree of interest in traditional cultural arts, dress, foods, sports, hobbies.

Psychological/somatic mindedness

Often there is an assumption that a clear dichotomy exists between the psychological and somatic perceptions of distress. This is a false dichotomy. The purpose for bearing this distinction in mind is to ascertain patients' ability to relate his symptoms in his own way; thus allowing some help in treatment recommendations; for example, whether physical or psychological therapies will be acceptable. Too often, the label of somatization is applied in a derogatory manner especially if there has been a poor communication.

Previous experience of services and treatment

Such information is helpful in any psychiatric assessment, since in working with patients from other cultures, previous bad experiences may deter the patient from using the services optimally. Previous experiences may not necessarily have occurred in this country and the criteria for help-seeking and service provisions may differ widely, thereby making acceptability of statutory services problematic.

Racial discrimination

Members from ethnic minorities are likely to have experienced discrimination in one or more fields of daily activities; for example, legal, financial, educational, or health care activities. This may be full-blown open discriminatory experience or suspected prejudicial treatment. This discriminatory behaviour could be on account of skin colour, religion, language, sex, race, or other factors which may well be masked under a broader umbrella. Do not underestimate the impact of such events and do not assume you understand the context. Ask about such events in a careful paced sensitive manner so that the patient may respond accordingly. Even if perceived racist experiences do not directly contribute to the patient's presentation treat such reports with respect and do not dismiss them as unimportant or irrelevant. If patients find that such experiences are not being understood or taken seriously, they may find it difficult to trust you with more sensitive information. Your attempts to focus away from these experiences on to only psychiatrically relevant issues will be sensed and interpreted as evidence of further power imbalance and could fracture a budding treatment alliance. Anyone who has been exposed to these experiences directly or indirectly is understandably sensitive to repeated trauma of this kind and may interpret an unsatisfactory assessment and consultation as discriminatory.

The limitation of the standard mental state examination

The standard mental health examination (MSE) must be as thorough and detailed as with any other patient. However, where the patient does not share the mental health professional's culture (regardless of skin colour) then any symptoms and signs must be appraised critically in a cultural context and the appraisal reviewed in response to emergence of more information. Various cultural, religious, and social groups are more likely to have varying and possibly unique idioms of distress, but to list them would suggest that clinicians could and should follow a recipe of cultural assessment based on the initial and perhaps erroneous impressions about the impact of cultural, religious, and social differences. However, application of diagnostic processes without due attention to socio-cultural influences is likely to meet with numerous pitfalls.

Behaviour

Behaviours which to the assessing clinician may appear odd or bizarre may have a culturally sanctioned role. For example, speaking in tongues, excessive religiosity, and trance possession, are culturally sanctioned in some cultures. These phenomena can only be evaluated by carefully recording the behaviour, the patient's explanation for it and the family and the cultural group's response to it. These views, if a sign of illness, may change as the patient recovers and become important signs by which the patients, their carers, and others in the folk sector may in the future identify a relapse. Unusual behaviour which is not clearly understandable is too readily assigned as evidence of psychosis without due attention to the adaptive/coping potential of the behaviour

Aggression

Aggression is often labelled as being a manifestation of psychosis. Potential aggression is especially difficult to anticipate and the interviewer may err on the side of caution by intervening too early if feeling threatened. Early intervention may well jeopardize any future treatment alliance. Our biology interacts with culturally shaped experiences to produce frustration and then to assert dominance and respond in a variety of ways, of which aggression is one. The only way to assess a potentially aggressive patient is to have no doubt about your safety. Ensure you are accompanied and encouraging a relative or friend of the patient to join you There may be cultural norms of frustration and conflict resolution. Do not be prompted to anticipate an aggressive situation through your own fear of assault from a patient with whom you do not share cultural values, norms, and mores.

Hallucinations

Check the patient's exact experiences. How consistent are they, and can they be differentiated from illusions and suggestibility states? If the patient uses figures of speech inexactly to articulate their experience of illness, do not erroneously identify them as hallucinations. The presence of visual phenomena are especially difficult to locate firmly within the standard framework of psycho-pathology.

Delusions

The traditional definition of delusion does take the role of culture and its context into account. There is, of course, a hypothetical possibility that if the examiner is not clear about the culture values that a delusional experience may be misattributed. Religious ideas, culturally sanctioned explanations, and spiritual or cosmic explanations, must be identified carefully and documented verbatim. Do not just record your impressions. Always consider alternative reasons for a patient's beliefs with their relatives or advocates. Again, record intact their responses. If a belief is culturally unfamiliar and is coupled with functional impairment or culturally inappropriate behaviour then its is likely to be a sign of illness.

First rank symptoms

World Health Organization studies have demonstrated the existence of core symptoms of schizophrenia across cultures. However, there is considerable concern that first-rank symptoms can occur in other psychiatric states and also in the course of culturally sanctioned methods of resolving distress (for example, passivity, possession, exorcism, delusions of control). Anecdotal evidence also suggests that some of the first-rank symptoms are best picked up if a patient's first or preferred language is used for interviewing.

Cognitive assessment

The standard cognitive assessment may yield very little diagnostic psychopathology if used blindly across cultures, especially with different languages. It is better to get third party information on memory failure and intellectual decline. If schedules of cognitive assessment are available in the patient's primary language these must be employed bearing in mind the patient's level of education and, once again, the help of an advocate or a team member who speaks the patient's first language can be invaluable.

Management

The management of patients from other cultures must be balanced with the patient's wishes. You may be making clinical decisions on the basis of information which is less than adequate; therefore, a careful risk assessment is warranted. Do not prescribe symptomatically if the diagnosis remains unclear. This will lead to false expectations on the part of the patient and may expose them to adverse side-effects that render them less inclined to return or take medication in the future.

If the problem is not urgent and there is sufficient time, arrange a further assessment time. This will allow you to think about the patient's presentation, and to obtain supervision and obtain corroborative information from past records, other health professionals, family members, etc., and it will also give you a further opportunity to garner information on the patient's culture. Let the patient know that you will be doing this.

Inferences

Be sure to discuss your inferences, diagnosis, and management plans with the patient, his advocates, or identified family members. The appropriateness of aetiological and diagnostic inferences should be considered with an awareness that such a process is influenced by culture. Your assumptions about these inferences should be checked with the patient. If the patient and other interested parties including advocates disagree with your intended management plan arrange to meet and discuss risk assessment. You should not alienate valuable community support otherwise your aftercare plans may be compromised or the community team may end up carrying a bigger level of involvement than possible.

Consultation dynamics

As discussed above, the patient's models of what the doctor does may be quite different from what you are able to offer. Some ethnic minorities will have a great respect for the health professions (doctors in particular), such that they may not confront, question, disagree, or point out the problems they may be facing. Although not a crisis, such a problem may manifest later as selective omission of medication, inaccurate reporting of symptoms, and consultation with other healers who may prove to be beneficial in the treatment of illness but may in some cases deter the patient from attending services or, more commonly, offer excessive reassurance or the promise of a miraculous cure which will encourage patients to disengage from the statutory sector.

Box 3.4 Good practice points

- Identify emotional idioms of distress and develop a shared vocabulary with the patient. Ask for clarification if symptoms or signs appear unusual or unfamiliar.

- Assume nothing about the patient. Do not be judgmental about patterns of communication or domination of the clinical interview by one family member — this may be cultural or the family style of communication.

- Be sensitive to the effects of your action, the setting or the referral mode which jeopardizes trust.

- Be sensitive to religious and social taboos.

- Discuss the findings with an independent person (perhaps an advocate) properly familiar with the culture within the bounds of strict confidentiality. Seek the patient's permission to do so.

- Explore the patient's capacity to take part in the consultation. Choose a consultation style and setting which is comfortable for the patient.

- Explore the family's language limitations, sense of urgency or crisis and realistic capacity for adopting strategies avaiblable to them, and making use of skills and strenghts — do not inadvertently undermine these.

4
The mental state examination

We will first consider mental state examinations of children (this page), then adults (p. 77), followed by special points during examinations of the elderly (p. 83) and those with learning disability (p. 86). Special aspects of the examination — neuropsychiatric assessment of both adults and children, examination of those with epilepsy, catatonia, or those who are mute or in a stupor will be found in the next chapter (pp. 113–19).

Children

The psychiatric interview with the child must serve several purposes. The mental state may provide additional information, as well as details of the history unavailable from other sources. It allows objective observations to be made that contribute to the diagnosis. The interview with the psychiatrist is also an event of considerable emotional significance to the child. Even if the child only attends once, that contact may have a considerable impact and it is important that it is therapeutically beneficial.

The reader is referred to Chapter 2 for a description of the preferred setting and for general advice, common errors, engagement as well as guides to interviewing children over and under 6 years of age.

Confidentiality

Confidentiality needs to be negotiated, particularly with adolescents. The procedure varies with the age and development of the child. The expectation is that the interview will be held in confidence. However, some secrets may have to be revealed to others.

At the end of an assessment interview it is good practice to clarify with the child whether there is anything they do not want mentioned. These confidences should be kept unless it is impossible, in which case this should be made explicit, for example: 'This is so serious I think your parents have to know about it — will you tell them or shall I?' If the child is being seen for a court report or social services assessment this should be made clear at the onset.

Scheme for a description of mental state

General description

- appearance, attractiveness, manner, style of dress, any evidence of neglect
- response to separation from parents, entering the interview room and the doctor's attempts to make contact.

Child's adjustment to the situation

- apprehension, appropriate or excessive reserve, emerging confidence, friendliness, disruption, age appropriateness
- topics of spontaneous conversation.

Motor activity

- amount of movement: reduced or increased
- co-ordination
- involuntary movements
- posturing
- rituals
- hyperventilation

If any problems are noted, fuller neurological evaluation is needed.

Language

- hearing: sounds, speech
- comprehension

- speech/vocalization/babble:
  - (a) spontaneity
  - (b) quantity, rate, and rhythm (e.g. stuttering)
  - (c) pattern of intonation and stress
  - (d) articulation: for example, dysarthria
  - (e) grammatical accuracy and complexity
  - (f) specific abnormalities, e.g. echoing, stereotyped features, I/you reversals (with written example if appropriate);
- gesture: imitation/comprehension/use.

  If any problems are noted, go to p. 41.

Social response to interviewer

- social responsiveness to examiners manner and comments, e.g. praise, reward
- rapport and eye contact: quality, quantity
- reciprocity and empathy
- social style; for example, reserved, shy, expansive
- disinhibited, cheeky, precocious, teasing
- negativistic, non-compliant, untruthful, surly
- ingratiating, manipulative

  If any problems are noted, go to p. 42.

Affect

- emotional expressiveness and range
- happiness
- anxiety: free-floating, situational, or specific phobias
- panic attacks
- observable tension
- signs of autonomic disturbance
- tearfulness

- sadness, wretchedness, despair, apathy
- thoughts of suicide or running away
- shame, embarrassment, perplexity
- anger, aggressiveness
- irritability.

Thought content

- worries, fears
- preoccupations, obsessions, suspicions
- hopelessness, guilt
- low self-esteem, self-hatred
- fantasies or wishes:
  - (a) spontaneously mentioned
  - (b) evoked (for example, 3 wishes)
- quality of ideation/play
- abnormal beliefs or experiences.

Cognition

- attention span/distractibility
- persistence
- curiosity
- orientation in time and space
- memory.

Attainment

Reading, spelling, and arithmetic are best assessed using standardized tests (for example, Neale and Schonell for reading). If a formal assessment by a psychologist is unavailable then the child should be asked to read simple passages, to recall their gist, and to write a sentence about a previous event. The fluency, accuracy, and comprehension of reading are all important. This testing is even more necessary for children showing disturbed behaviour or frustration in the classroom.

Standardized measures

Increasing numbers of rating scales for parents and teachers are available, and standardized structured or semi-structured interviews are used for some clinical purposes.

Advantages of explicit and formalized interviewing schemes are that they ensure a systematic cover of key parts, and can provide standards as to whether a problem is severe enough to be deviant. A corresponding disadvantage is that they cannot cover everything. The crucial aspect of an individual case may be uncommon or even unique. Standardized schemes may divert attention away from the individually significant to what is common. They need to be supplemented with the general clinical enquiry described here. Most symptoms in child psychiatry are on a continuum with normality. The judgement of what constitutes a disorder should be based not only on the levels of symptoms, but also on an assessment of their impact on child and family.

Rating scales for parents and teachers are valuable as group tests, and sometimes for screening purposes. However, they are not yet sufficiently sensitive or specific for diagnosing an individual child. Rater effects, as well as the child's behaviour, will determine how they are completed.

Interviewer's subjective response to child

Conclusion

Finally, an opinion should be expressed on whether (and how) the child's mental state departs from the expected in relation to age, IQ, sex, and social background.

Adults

The description of the patient's mental state should 'record behavioural and psychological data elicited by examination at the time of the interview *as well as observations made in the ward and other parts of the hospital*. There are three aspects to interviewing — obtaining information, observing the patient in a two-person interaction, and giving support. The areas of information that need to be covered in the mental state examination are detailed below. The opportunity should also be taken to record the way the patient reacts to the interviewer and how the interviewer feels. For people with learning disability whose major disability is significant but not severe, the normal mental state examination can be applied.

When describing the mental state of a patient, even very briefly, the term 'normal' is usually inappropriate. Some factual information should be given under as many of the listed headings as possible, so that a clinical judgement can be made of its significance. Such information may also be very useful for future reference.

Appearance and general behaviour

Give as complete, accurate, and lifelike a description as possible of how the patient appears and what can be observed in their behaviour: way of spending the day, eating, sleep, cleanliness in general, self-care, hair, cosmetics, dress; behaviour towards other patients, doctors and nursing staff. Is the patient relaxed or tense and restless; slow, hesitant, or repetitive? Do movements and attitudes have an apparent purpose or meaning? How does the patient respond to various requirements and situations? Are there abnormal responses to external events? Can his attention be held and diverted? Does the patient appear frightened? Does he appear frightening? (see p. 132.)

Does the patient's behaviour suggest that he is disorientated? Specify orientation if doubtful. Describe gestures, grimaces, and other motor expressions. Is there much or little activity? Does it vary during the day, is it spontaneous, or how is it provoked? Does the patient, if inactive, resist passive movements, or maintain an attitude, obey commands, or indicate awareness at all? Do hallucinations seem to modify his behaviour? Even if the patient does not speak, there should still be a full and careful report of his posture and behaviour.

Talk

The **form** of the patient's utterances rather than their content is considered here. Does he say much or little, talk spontaneously or only in answer, slowly or quickly, hesitantly or promptly, to the point or wide of it, coherently, anxiously, discursively, loosely with interruptions, with sudden silences, with frequent changes of topic, commenting on events and things at hand, appropriately, using strange words or syntax, rhymes, puns? How does the form of his talk vary with its subject? Attach or include in the notes any abnormal written productions. A *verbatim sample of talk should be recorded at this point if there are abnormalities of form.* It should give an adequate demonstration of formal disorders of thinking such as flight of ideas, thought block, disorder of logical association, reiterations, perseveration, incoherence, neologisms, paraphasias, etc.

Mood

The patient's appearance, motility, posture, and general behaviour, as described above, may give some indication of his mood. In addition, answers to questions such as 'How do you feel in yourself?', 'What is your mood?', 'How about your spirits?', or some similar inquiry should be recorded. Whenever depressive mood is suspected specific enquiry should be made about the following: tearfulness; diurnal variation of mood; suicidal ideas or plans; attitude to the future; self-esteem; guilt; appetite; weight; and libido. Many variations of mood may be present, not merely happiness or sadness, namely such states as anxiety, fear, suspicion, perplexity, and others which it is convenient to include under this heading. Observe the constancy of the mood during the interview, the influences which change it and the appropriateness of the patient's apparent emotional state to what he says. Note evidence of flatness or lability of affect, and specify any indications that the patient is concealing his true feelings.

Thought content

This should include morbid thoughts and preoccupations. The patient's answers to questions such as 'What do you see as your main worries?' should be summarized. Are there anxieties or pre-occupations with the present life situation, with the future, with the past, with the safety of the self or others? Do worries interfere with concentration or sleep? Are there any phobias or obsessional ruminations, compulsions, or rituals?

Abnormal beliefs and interpretations of events

Specify the content, mode of onset and degree of fixity of any abnormal beliefs.

- in relation to the environment, e.g. ideas of reference, mis-interpretations or delusions; beliefs that he is being persecuted, that he is being treated in a special way, or is the subject of an experiment
- in relation to the body; for example, ideas or delusions of bodily change.
- in relation to the self; for example, delusions of passivity, influence, thought reading, or intrusion.

Abnormal experiences referred to environment, body, or self

Environment: Hallucinations and illusions — auditory, visual, olfactory, gustatory, or tactile; feelings of familiarity or unfamil-iarity; derealization; *déjà-vu*.

Body: Feelings of deadness, pain, or other alterations of bodily sensation, somatic hallucinations.

Self: Depersonalization, awareness of disturbance in mechanism of thinking, or blocking or retardation, autochthonous ideas, etc.

The source, content, vividness, reality, and other characteristics of these experiences should be recorded, and also the time of occurrence; for example, at night, when alone, when falling asleep, or awakening.

The cognitive state

This should be briefly assessed in every patient and related to his general intelligence (see p. 82). In younger patients where cerebral organic disease is not suspected, the tests mentioned in the following notes for orientation, attention and concentration, as well as memory should be administered. For older patients see the section on assessment of the elderly patient (p. 83). However, when cognitive impairment or cerebral disease is suspected, further tests will need to be administered from the schema for the further examination of patients with suspected organic cerebral disease (Chapter 5, pp. 91–7).

Orientation

If there is any reason to doubt the patient's orientation, record their answers to questions about their own name and identity, the place where they are, the time of day, and the date.

Attention and concentration

Is the patient's attention easily aroused and sustained? Does he concentrate? Is he easily distracted? To test for concentration and attention, ask him to tell you the days or the months in reverse order, or to do simple arithmetical problems requiring 'carrying over' (for example 112–25) or subtraction of serial 7s from 100 (give answers and time taken). Give the patient digits to repeat forwards, and then others to repeat backwards (delivered evenly and at one-second intervals) and record how many can be reproduced in each direction.

Memory

In all cases memory should be assessed by comparing the patient's account of his life with that given by others, and by examining his account for intrinsic evidence of gaps or inconsistencies. Special attention should be paid to memory for recent events, such as his admission to hospital and happenings in the ward since. Where there is selective impairment of memory for special incidents, periods, or recent or remote happenings this should be recorded in detail, and the patient's attitude to his forgetfulness and the things forgotten especially investigated. Record any evidence of confabulation or false memories. If the patient confabulates, is this spontaneous or in response to suggestion only? Retrograde and anterograde amnesia must be specified in detail in relation to head injury or epileptic phenomena.

If there is any suspicion of impairment of memory, record verbatim the patient's attempt to repeat a name and address or other similar data immediately and 5 minutes later.

The following task provides the opportunity for testing free and cued recall separately, and will sometimes demonstrate good learning ability when other techniques have failed. It may also reveal perseveration or confabulation. The patient is told he will be given the name of a flower and asked to repeat it ('the flower is — a daffodil — please repeat daffodil'), then a colour ('the colour — is blue — please repeat blue'), then a town ('the town is — Brighton — please repeat Brighton'), etc. The list continues with items such as cars, days of the week etc., until six to ten items have been given according to the patient's ability. Recall is tested 3–5 minutes later, first without prompting, then, if necessary, after repeating each category name.

Intelligence

The patient's expected intelligence should be gauged from his history, his general knowledge, and his educational and occupational record. Where this is unknown simple tests for general information and grasp should be given, and an assessment made of his experience and interests. An indirect measure of intelligence might also be obtained from assessing the patient's scholastic achievements by testing his reading, spelling, and arithmetical abilities. A more objective measure can be obtained using the Mill Hill and Progressive Matrices Tests from which an Intelligence Quotient (IQ) can be derived. A learning disorder should be suspected if a discrepancy is found between the results of these' tests and the level of intelligence anticipated by assessing the patient's literacy and numeracy.

Patient's appraisal of illness, difficulties, and prospects

What is the patient's attitude to his present state? Does he regard it as an illness, as 'physical', 'mental', or 'nervous', or as needing treatment? What does he attribute it to? Is he aware of mistakes made spontaneously or in response to tests? How does he regard these and other details of his condition? How does he regard previous experiences, mental illnesses, etc.? Can he appreciate possible connections between his illness and stressful life situations, spontaneously or when suggested? Are his attitudes constructive or unconstructive, realistic or unrealistic? Is his judgement good when discussing financial or domestic problems, etc.? What does he propose to do when he has left the hospital? What is his attitude to supervision and care?

The interviewer's reaction to the patient

Here a brief account should be given of the way in which the interviewer is affected by the patient's behaviour. Did the patient arouse sympathy, concern, sadness, anxiety, irritation, frustration, impatience, or anger? Did the interviewer find it easy or difficult to control any untoward responses evoked in him or has he failed to do so and, if so, how?

The elderly

Some elderly patients with dementia are unwilling to undergo formal testing and respond with irritation, unexplained refusal, or bland replies such as: 'I don't pay attention to that sort of thing'. Such replies are sometimes an attempt to camouflage an impairment and should be handled with tact and discretion. If the patient persists in refusing to answer, the interviewer might attempt to engage in neutral conversation, noting any internal inconsistencies in the patient's responses which might indicate cognitive impairment.

Where the patient permits formal testing the use of a short cognitive screening test such as the Abbreviated Mental Test or the Mini-mental State Examination should be performed (see below). In addition, tests of parietal and frontal lobe function should be carried out (see pp. 93–7).

Mood state

Some elderly patients with profound depression deny depressed mood but show other prominent symptoms such as anxiety, somatic or dissociative symptoms, or cognitive impairment.

Psychotic and behavioural problems

These are best elicited from an informant.

Physical examination

Many elderly patients suffer from concurrent physical illness, and a thorough physical examination should always be carried out. Special attention should be given to any signs of physical trauma, possibly occurring as a result of abuse.

Environment

If the patient is being assessed at home some inspection of the home environment should be made. This is an important part in evaluating the degree of risk posed to the patient (and possibly others). Remember that self-neglect is not diagnostic of any particular disorder and can occur in severe functional illness as well as dementia.

- Is the dwelling in a good state of repair and decoration?
- Is it secure?
- Are the gas, electricity, and water supplies connected?
- Is there adequate heating and lighting?
- Is the gas ever left on unlit?

- If the patient smokes, is there evidence of the careless use of lighted cigarettes?
- Is the patient able to call for help if necessary (e.g. via a centralized alarm system)?
- Is there enough food in the home to make, at least, small snacks/hot drinks?
- Is there evidence of urinary or faecal incontinence?
- Are any pets well-cared for?

Abbreviated Mental Test Score (AMTS) (see Table 4.1)

This is derived from the Blessed Mental Test Score[3] and is widely used in assessing elderly patients particularly in general practice and geriatric medicine. A score of 6/10 or less is indicative of

Table 4.1 Abbreviated Mental Test Score (AMTS)
Instruction: score one point for each question answered correctly.

Question

1 How old are you?	.....
2 What time is it now (to the nearest hour)?	.....
Give address to be recalled at the end of the test:	
for example, 42 West Street.	
3 What is the name of the hospital	
(or area of town, if at home)?	
1.....	
4 What year is it now?	.....
5 What date were you born?	.....
6 What month is it now?	.....
7 What were the dates of the First World War?	.....
8 What is the name of the Monarch (or President in USA)?	.....
9 Please count backwards from 20 to 1	
(no errors allowed, but may correct self).	.....
10 What was the address I asked you to remember?	.....
Total	

cognitive impairment. It has no advantage over the Mini-mental State Examination (MMSE), other than being briefer.

Mini-Mental State Examination (MMSE)

This test was developed at the Johns Hopkins University for use in neurological patients, but it has since been validated in a wide variety of settings. A score of 23 or less is indicative of 'dementia'. The MMSE is sensitive to the effects of age, educational background, and socio-economic status. For patients over 70 years of age who left school before they were 15, the cut point should be reduced by 3 points, see Appendix 1, p. 243.

People with learning disability

Mild or moderate learning disability

By definition, a learning-disabled person will have a degree of developmental delay. Detailed examination of the mental state is critical: this is not easy, but much information can be gained by observation.

Mood disorders and psychoses may present initially as behavioural changes: for example, overactivity in hypomania; social withdrawal in depression. Autistically disabled people usually become more inaccessible when depressed: they present as 'more autistic'.

Abnormal mental phenomena may be expressed in a fleeting and fragmentary manner: sustained observation is often necessary to allow any abnormalities to emerge. Do not waste time looking for specific syndromes.

Severe learning difficulties

Severely mentally handicapped people may demonstrate a major communication impairment. It is, therefore, necessary to eliminate pain or a physical illness as the precipitant of a behavioural crisis. The first sign of a developing physical or mental illness may be an exacerbation of pre-existing symptoms or behaviour. For example, at the onset of a mood disorder in an autistic person, there may initially be just an exaggeration of the autistic features. Pre-existing handicap (for instance a speech impediment) may mask the expression of typical mental symptoms. In this case, check for secondary symptoms, for example, vegetative features (sleep, appetite, weight, etc.) when depression is suspected. The mental state may be difficult to define in detail, in which case the diagnosis must be based upon a balance of probabilities.

Remember: all clinical notes should be signed and dated.

5
Neuropsychiatric assessment and epilepsy

Neuropsychiatric assessment

History

This usually provides the diagnosis; examination should be considered confirmatory.

Presenting complaint

When was a change first noticed? Who noticed it first? How did it affect daily function? What was the reason for presentation to the general practitioner? What was the effect of any intervention at that stage? Were there any precipitating or relieving factors? A

Table 5.1 Time course and diagnosis of neuropsychiatric disease

Rapid decline and complete recovery	Transient ischaemic attack, epilepsy, transient global amnesia
Slow steady decline	Alzheimer's disease, Huntington's disease, Parkinson's disease, normal-pressure hydrocephalus
Rapid steady decline	Encephalitis, brain tumour, raised intracranial pressure, cerebral abscess
Stepwise deterioration	Vascular dementia, multiple sclerosis
Diurnal variation	Myasthenia gravis
Static condition	Autism, Asperger's syndrome, cerebral palsy

time course of the disorder is most helpful in aiding the diagnosis of neuropsychiatric disease (Table 5.1).

Collateral history from an informant is crucial in confirming the onset and course of the disorder, particularly when there is a suspicion of cognitive impairment or clouding of consciousness. This means telephone interviewing the family, friends, work colleagues, as well as discussion with nursing staff following the patient's admission to hospital.

Family history

Is there a history of fits, memory problems, dementia, or nervous trouble?

Personal history

Ask about:

- of delayed walking/talking or other milestones?
- Any learning difficulties?
- Educational attainment?
- Promotions or later decline at work?
- Any occupational hazards, e.g. lead or solvents?
- Amount, frequency, mode of administration (such as IV) of recreational drugs consumed, including alcohol, pattern of consumption over time.

Previous medical history (Table 5.2)

Enquire for childhood infections, fits, or head injury. Has the patient ever lost consciousness: how long and what memory blanks before and after; has the patient ever seen a neurologist or physician?

Prescribed medication (Table 5.3)

Has the patient ever suffered any side-effects?

Table 5.2 Previous medical history suggesting organic cause

Epilepsy	Postictal/ictal/interictal psychosis, Todd's paresis
Head injury	Acute/chronic subdural, alcohol abuse
Connective tissue disease	Dementia, depression, psychosis
Thyroid disease	Anxiety, depression, dementia
Diabetes	Hypoglycaemic episodes, cerebrovascular events, dementia
Cardiovascular disease	Hypoxic delirium, sleep apnoea
Surgery/anaesthetic	Cognitive impairment from hypoxic episodes
Sepsis	Brain abscess
Menstrual disturbance	Pituitary adenoma
Urinary incontinence	Frontal syndrome, normal-pressure hydrocephalus

The examination

This begins when the patient enters the room. Do not hurry the patient and note the degree of co-operation. If cognitive impairment seems present move to a full cognitive examination rather than struggle to obtain the history. If there is an apparent decreased level of consciousness, monitor this by using the Glasgow coma scale (best verbal and motor responses, and pupillary reflex).

Cognitive examination

Keep in mind premorbid intelligence.

Orientation

Does the patient know who they are, where they are, and what the date is?

Table 5.3 Drugs contributing to neuropsychiatric disorder

Neuroleptics (except clozapine), antiemetics	Movement disorders
Lithium	Tremor, confusion, ataxia
Neuroleptics	Neuroleptic Malignant Syndrome (pyrexia, rigidity, autonomic lability, decreased consciousness)
SSRIs, MAOIs, TCAs, lithium	Serotonin syndrome (restlessness, altered mental state, hyperreflexia, tremor, fits, rigors, myoclonus)
Amphetamines, appetite suppressants	Anxiety, insomnia, psychosis
Steroids	Confusion, depression, psychosis
Benzodiazepines	Dependence, confusional state, ataxia, withdrawal syndrome
LSD, cocaine	Psychosis
Alcohol	Dependence, withdrawal syndrome, Wernicke–Korsakoff syndrome, ataxia, peripheral neuropathy, decreased consciousness, dementia, head injury, acute/chronic subdural
Antiepileptics	Confusion, ataxia, psychosis (especially vigabatrin)

Attention and concentration

Can the patient give months of the year backwards or spell 'world' backwards? Or subtract 7s serially from 100? Make a note of the number of errors and don't confront the patient with their mistakes! 'Digit span recall' tests concentration; a forward span of five or more is considered normal. Remember to deliver each digit in a monotone one-second apart.

Memory

Often separated into immediate recall, **short-term memory** (STM), and **long-term memory** (LTM). Normal practice is to test

semantic memory by name and address recall; an address local to the patient is usually chosen. The patient is asked to repeat the full name and address immediately (**registration**). If one or more mistakes are made then the entire name and address should be provided again. Conventionally this continues for five attempts, at which point the simpler three-object recall method can be employed. The three objects should be categorically different; for example, apple, table, penny.

Recall (STM)

This is tested after 5 or 10 minutes, and the number of errors recorded. Each word or number contributes to the final score. Problems with retrieval rather than storage can be discerned by providing a choice of approximate alternatives to the item forgotten. Anxiety is the most common cause of retrieval failure.

Long term memory difficulties (LTM)

LTM should be apparent from the history, and the informant.

Non-verbal memory

This should be assessed by asking the patient to reproduce a simple figure such as a Saxon cross or a clock-face showing a specific time, after a 5-minute interval. Initial copying of the figure tests **constructional praxis** (see below), as well as registration.

Apraxia

Apraxia is the inability to perform a volitional act even though the peripheral motor system and sensorium are intact. **Constructional apraxia** has been tested by the drawing above. **Dressing apraxia** (said to be a non-dominant parietal lobe problem) is evident from the informant or by asking the patient to dress. **Gait apraxia** is assessed by the tandem gait test (see below). **Ideomotor apraxia** is usually tested by giving the patient a three-stage command, for example: 'Touch your left ear with your right ring finger and then point to the window'.

Agnosia

Here the problem is the inability to understand the significance of sensory stimuli even though the sensory pathways and sensorium

Table 5.4 Features of parietal lobe dysfunction

Dominant	Dysphasia	Receptive dysphasia
	Gerstmann's syndrome[1]	Finger agnosia, dyscalculia, R/L disorientation, agraphia
Non-dominant	Topographical disorientation[2]	Getting lost, inability to learn new routes
	Visuospatial agnosia[2]	Inability to recognize from visually presented information
	Constructional apraxia[2]	Difficulty in copying visually presented model, e.g. 3D cube
	Anosognosia[2]	Failure to recognize a disabled limb
	Prosopagnosia[2]	Inability to recognize faces (associated with posterior lesion)
	Neglect[2]	Patient pays no attention to one side; for example, by shaving one side of face, drawing clock with only half represented

[1] More often seen in Multiple choice questions than clinically.
[2] Not very well lateralized, but deficits more common and severe with right hemisphere damage.

Table 5.5 Associated neurological deficit with parietal lesions

Optic radiation	Homonymous lower quadrantanopia
Sensory cortex	Contralateral disturbance, such as astereognosis, reduced discrimination
Perceptual rivalry	Visual and sensory inattention

are intact. **Astereognosia** is the failure to identify three-dimensional form and is tested by placing a familiar object in the patient's hand, for example a key. **Visual agnosia** is assessed by asking the patient to perform a command which is written down (assuming they can read); for example; 'Close your eyes'. **Agraphognosia** (or **agraphaesthesia**) is detected by tracing

Table 5.6 Features of temporal lobe dysfunction

Dominant	Receptive dysphasia	Including alexia and agraphia in posterior lesions
	Memory disturbance	Especially for verbal material
Non-dominant	Visuospatial deficits[1]	For example, object and face recognition
	Amusia	Difficulty with melody, cadence, and emotional content of music
	Memory disturbance	Especially for non-verbal material

[1] Not well lateralized, but deficits more common and severe with right hemisphere damage.

Table 5.7 Associated neurological deficits with temporal lobe lesions

Auditory cortex	Cortical deafness
Optic radiation	Homonymous upper quadrantanopia
Bilateral medial temporal lobe	Amnesic syndromes
Limbic system	Personality changes–depersonalization, emotional instability, aggressive or antisocial behaviour

numbers on the palms with a retracted ball-point pen which the patient then fails to recognize.

Language ability

Dysarthria, a difficulty in the mechanical production of speech, should be assessed before **dysphasia**, which is the cortical partial failure of language function. Asking the patient to repeat a difficult phrase such as 'West Register Street' will elicit dysarthria.

Expressive dysphasia can be tested by asking the patient to name everyday objects such as a pen or watch and parts thereof

Table 5.8 Features of frontal lobe dysfunction

Social behaviour	Disinhibition, distractability, slowed psychomotor activity[1]
Motivation, planning, and initiating	Lack of drive,[1] poor goal setting, and learning
Organizing and problem solving	Errors of judgement, failure to anticipate, perseveration[1]
Adapting and shifting attention	Catastrophic response,[1] inability to adapt to the unexpected[1]
Personality	Over-familiarity, tactlessness, empty fatuous euphoria,[1] sexual indiscretion

[1] Characteristics which help differentiate from mania.

Table 5.9 Associated neurological deficit with frontal lesions

Broca's area	Expressive dysphasia if dominant hemisphere
Precentral gyrus motor complex	Contralateral hemiplegia
Supplementary motor area	Paralysis of head and eye movement (head and eyes turn towards diseased side) present only in the acute stage of a lesion, compensation occurring after a few days
Paracentral lobule	Bowel and bladder dysfunction
Optic nerve	Ipsilateral optic atrophy (when associated with contralateral papilloedema = Foster–Kennedy syndrome)
Olfactory nerve	Anosmia

(**nominal dysphasia**). They can also be asked to write a brief passage to dictation and a sentence of their own choice. **Receptive dysphasia** can be detected by asking the patient to read and explain a passage of appropriate difficulty, as well as getting them to respond to verbal commands.

'Tests' of frontal lobe function

The validity and reliability of these is *not* beyond dispute. **Verbal fluency** is the ability to generate categorical lists, for example ask the patient to name as many 4-legged animals as possible in the next minute, or words beginning with the letter 'T' in 1 minute. Normal is above 15. This is said to be a dominant lobe function. **Motor sequencing,** such as the fist-edge–palm test, should be assessed by first demonstrating the sequence to the patient and then asking them to continue the imitation for at least 30 seconds. Remember to vary the sequence between left and right hands to avoid a learning effect. Remember that anxiety is the most common cause of errors.

Traditionally, **abstract reasoning** is evaluated by proverb interpretation. Start by asking the meaning of a simple proverb such as: 'People in glass houses shouldn't throw stones', and progress to

Table 5.10   Other less common frontal lobe tests

Primitive reflexes	Grasp	Grasping of the contralateral hand when stroking the palm from the radial to ulnar side
	Pout	Pouting of the lips, elicited by either stroking down the filtrum or by gently tapping on a spatula placed over the lips
	Palmomental	A 'wince' on stroking the ipsilateral thenar eminence
Alternate tapping		Ability to understand a simple tapped code and adapt when told that the rules have changed, e.g. ABABAB–AABBAABB
Perseveration		Motor or verbal; inability to avoid repeating the last given action or word
Reciprocal co-ordination		Ability to use both hands simultaneously smoothly and quickly without example
Cognitive estimates		e.g. How many camels in Holland? How tall is the Post Office tower?

more complex ones, for example: 'A rolling stone gathers no moss'.

Occipital lobe lesions

These can lead to simple or complex visual hallucinations, as well as difficulties with visual recognition.

Lesions in the brainstem

Lesions here or in other midline structures, such as the dien-cephalon, can lead to hypersomnia, 'akinetic mutism', or an amnestic syndrome. Mood disturbance and intellectual decline have also been reported.

Neurological examination

The examination does not have to be arduous for either the doctor or the patient. A recommended neuropsychiatric screen is given below, rather than a formal head-to-toe neurological examination. Note **handedness** by watching the patient write; right/left dis-crimination has already been assessed (see ideomotor apraxia). **Gait** is a good way of testing voluntary movement. Ask the patient to walk one foot in front of another, as though on a tightrope (**tandem gait test**)

Sitting or other resting posture allows the observation of involun-tary movements.

Reflexes can be quickly tested with a tendon hammer once the patient is sitting or recumbent. Hyperreflexic tendon jerks are most commonly due to anxiety. An upgoing (positive) plantar or

Babinski reflex indicates an upper motor neurone lesion. The primitive reflexes are described in Table 5.10.

Testing of **power** and **sensation** may be performed if the history indicates a deficit. Peripheral neuropathy is probably the most common positive finding, and may be due to diabetes, alcohol or lead poisoning.

    Cranial nerve testing, see Table 5.13.

Table 5.11 Assessing stance and gait

Deficit	Appearance	Confirmatory signs	Neuropsychiatric associations
Hemiplegic	Arm and hand flexed and internally rotated	Increased tone, brisk reflexes, upgoing plantar	Depression is common post CVA (especially in anterior lesions?). Hemiplegias acquired in childhood may lead to preserved language function at the expense of visuospatial skills, regardless of lesion site.
Parkinsonian	Stooped posture, reduced arm swing, bradykinesia, shuffling gait which improves with afferent input (e.g. walking with a friend)	'Lead pipe' rigidity, 'pill rolling' tremor which combine to give 'cogwheeling'. Paucity of speech and facial expression	Drug induced (where tremor uncommon) seen more than Parkinson's disease (PD). Personality change (obsessionality and hypochondriasis) said to characterize PD. Dementia:10–15%; depression common but unrelated to stage of disease. Psychosis usually iatrogenic.
Cerebellar	Wide-based stance and gait, slurred speech	Dysmetria (past pointing), intention tremor, nystagmus	Possible current intoxication (alcohol, lithium; anticonvulsants) or chronic damage (for example MS — look for pale discs, pyramidal signs) or alcoholism
Akathisia	Motor restlessness, inability to sit or stand still	Subjective sense of inner distress and motor tension	Present in 20–30% of patients on Neuroleptics, often overlooked

Table 5.12 Assessing abnormal movements

Deficit	Appearance	Confirmatory signs	Neuropsychiatric associations
Choreiform	Rapid, irregular dance-like or jerky involuntary movements	Consider more detailed cognitive testing	Accompanying medical condition, e.g. SLE, pregnancy, thyrotoxicosis. Drug-induced neuroleptics, phenytoin, the oral contraceptive pill (OCP, Basal ganglia vascular disease, neuroacanthocytosis, Huntington's disease
Tic disorders	Repeated jerky movements, mimicking normal actions and under some voluntary control	Ask about suppressibility, and obsessive compulsive phenomena	Common in children, but reduce with age. Usually affect periocular muscles, face, neck, and shoulders. Gilles de la Tourette syndrome begins with simple tics, progressing to jumps, genuflexions, and hops. Vocal tics and coprolalia also seen later
Dystonic	Sustained muscular contractions cause repetitive twisting movements, or abnormal postures and bizarre gaits. May occur focally, e.g. writer's cramp; spasmodic torticollis	Recheck medication history: neuroleptics; antiemetics; SSRIs; and lithium have been implicated	Acute dystonia rapidly relieved by anticholinergics. Tardive dystonia is difficult to treat and can be very disabling. Rarer causes include Wilson's disease (look for associated basal ganglia and liver disease) and Huntington's disease

Table 5.13 Assessing cranial nerve abnormalities

	Name	Testing	Importance
I	Olfactory	Omit — can be asked about	May be impaired in Alzheimer's disease or frontal lobe lesions
II	Optic	Ask re. acuity. Test fields by confrontation, both eyes at the same time: 'Which finger is wiggling?' Assess pupillary reaction to light and examine disks for swelling or atrophy	Important to detect a field defect as this may aid localization (see above). Hemianopia implies a contralateral hemisphere lesion. If visual inattention present (simultaneous finger wiggling) check parietal lobe function
III, IV, and VI	Oculomotor, trochlear, and abducens	Ask patient to follow your finger slowly, left to right, up and down. Look to either side on command. Ask re. diplopia	Opthalmoplegias are part of Wernicke's encephalopathy. IIIrd nerve (eye down and out) and VIth nerve (eye cannot abduct) palsies seen post-head injury. Acute IIIrd lesion suggests raised intracranial pressure
V	Trigeminal	Test sensation left and right on mandible, maxilla, and forehead. Ask patient to clench their jaw	Trigeminal neuralgia can occur after herpes zoster infection, and the excruciating pain can lead to suicide. Palliate with carbamazepine or antidepressants

Table 5.13 (*Continued*)

	Name	Testing	ImportanceI
VII	Facial	Observe facial symmetry	Beware paucity of facial expression in depression and Parkinsonism
VIII	Auditory	No need to test formally	Congenital rubella may result in deafness (plus cataract and low IQ)
IX and X	Glossopharyngeal and vagus	Listen to the voice and inspect the palate as the patient says 'Ah'	Lesion here (lower motor neurone) results in a bulbar palsy which may be due to tumour; Motor neurone disease; myasthenia gravis, etc. Pseudobulbar palsy (bilateral upper motor neurone lesion deafferenting the bulbar nuclei)
XI	Spinal accessory nerve	Ask patient to shrug their shoulders	
XII	Hypoglossal	Inspect tongue at rest, ask patient to stick out tongue	leads to dysarthria, a slow tongue, and a brisk jaw jerk. Often accompanied by emotional lability and a gait apraxia (marche á petit pas).

Reference: Kopelman, M.D. (1994). Structured psychiatric interview: assessment of the cognitive state. *British Journal Hospital Medicine*, **52**, 277–81.

Neurological screening examination of children over 5 years of age

Children with known physical conditions or a history suggestive of a physical condition (for example, epilepsy) should be given a full neurological examination rather than this short screen.

1. Inspect ordinary gait.
2. Ask child to mimic:
   (a) heel–toe walking;
   (b) tiptoe walking (possible above 3 years, usually no associated movements above 8 years);
   (c) hopping on each leg (hopping begins at 3–4 years);
   (d) kicking a ball of paper.
3. Inspection, particularly of hands and face, for dysmorphic features, etc.
4. Touch fingers in turn with thumb. Test finger–thumb co-ordination bilaterally. (Most 6- and some 5-year-olds can do it. Mirror movements usually absent after 10 years).
5. Check for dysdiadochokinesis on rapidly alternating hand movements (pronation/supination 15 seconds each side).
6. Touch my finger. Repeat three times for each hand (possible above 3 years, with eyes shut above 7 years). Note tremor, consistent deviation.
7. Stand up, arms out, fingers spread for 20 seconds. Age 4 upwards: look for choreiform (small, jerky, irregular) movements of fingers. Over age 6: eyes closed, mouth open, tongue out. Look for asymmetry and drift.
8. Close inspection of eyes including ocular movements. Visual fields to confrontation.
9. Check face and jaw movements and power — whistle, smile, blow out your cheeks. Note tongue movements, wiggle tongue, lick upper lip.
10. Child removes shoes and socks (check shoes for uneven wear):
    (a) check muscle power and tone in arms and legs;
    (b) check tendon and plantar reflexes;

(c) check feet for dysmorphic features;

(d) measure head circumference and plot on percentile chart;

(e) measure height and weight and plot on percentile chart;

(f) estimate pubertal status (Tanner stages described on reverse of percentile charts).

(g) Observe how child puts socks and shoes back on.

11. Test hearing:

(a) name large toy at 1 metre distance in a quiet voice (laryngeal component) — ball, doll, car, spoon, fork, brick, ship — out of the child's field of vision.

12. Check visual acuity (well-lit Snellen charts).

If abnormalities are detected a complete medical history should be taken and a full neurological examination given.

Epilepsy in children

The history

Begin by asking for details of the child's first attack: age, circumstances, description, duration, how it was dealt with. Then obtain similar details about subsequent attacks.

Be careful to distinguish and obtain separate descriptions of all different kinds of attack experienced. For each type of attack probe for points described in the following sections.

Pre-ictal

Precipitating events
Are they through: physical causes, illness, fever, etc.; psychological, any stress, or disturbance?

Timing
Do they occur at any particular time of the day or night, how long since the last meal, etc.?

Altered behaviour or mental state before fit
Is the patient irritable, restless, confused, apathetic, etc. — minutes or hours before the attack?

Patient's activity at onset
Do they occur while asleep, on wakening, or in full consciousness? Are they precipitated by overbreathing, watching TV, walking out into bright sun, or any other change?

Ictal

Aura
What are the patient's subjective, warning experiences? Ask the child whether they know the seizure is coming and what they notice first (giddiness, noises, lights, smell, funny taste, inability to speak, feels frightened, etc.). If the child cannot describe this experience they may be able to draw it.

Course
What is the first event noticed (noises, strange behaviour, cry, fall to ground, motionless stare, etc.)?

Posture during attack
Did the child fall, go limp, remain standing, slump back in chair, etc.?

Movements
Which parts moved? One side or both? Synchronous or not (for example, turning of head or eyes, tonic stiffening movements, clonic jerking movements, restless or semi-purposive behaviour, automatic or repetitive acts, fumbling, mouth movements)?

Spread (march) of movements
Where did the fit start? Did it spread anywhere?

Consciousness
Was the child totally unresponsive? Aware, but unable to talk? Fully conscious and talking?

Colour changes
Did the child become pale, flushed, or blue?

Autonomic effects
Examples include becoming hot and sweaty, cold and sweaty, or salivating.

Incontinence
Was there any incontinence of urine or faeces?

Injury
Was the tongue bitten or any other injury sustained?

Post-ictal

After-effects
Did they return to normal immediately or go to sleep or become sleepy? Were they confused? Was there any weakness or paralysis of arms or legs? Clumsiness? Difficulty with speech? Change of behaviour or emotional state? Other symptoms for example, headache, vomiting?

Duration and frequency of this type of fit

If these are not mentioned by the parent ask specifically regarding the following:

- *Generalized convulsive seizures*: for example, are there ever attacks in which they pass out completely? Are there movements of the arms or legs in any of these attacks — tonic/clonic or clonic/tonic/clonic?

- *Generalized absence seizures*: for example, is there ever a momentary blank spell in which they seem to be out of touch for a moment, but do not fall down, and for which there is no memory subsequently? Are there any movements at all whilst this is happening?

- *Other generalized attacks*: for example, do they ever show odd jerky movements (myoclonus)? Do they ever fall down suddenly without jerking or going stiff (drop attacks)?

- *Simple partial seizures*: for example, are there any attacks in which there are movements of the arms or legs, but the child does not pass out or lose touch?

- *Complex partial seizures*: for example, do they ever have episodes in which they do not seem themselves or do peculiar things?

- *Reflex attacks*: for example, do they know how to stop an attack coming on? Ask the child privately if he or she knows how to make an attack start.

Treatment

Is this prescribed by the family doctor or paediatrician? Which drugs are used and in what doses? (Calculate dose kg^{-1} day^{-1} — does it fall within the recommended range?) What side-effects are there? Have blood levels been measured recently? What do parents do during the attack?

Attitudes

Obtain parental attitude to the attacks. What did they think was happening during the first attack? What do they put them down to? What does the child put them down to?

Does the child have epilepsy?

- *Differential diagnosis*: includes syncope, breath-holding attacks, sleep disorder, benign paroxysmal vertigo.

- *Pseudo-seizures*: are more common in children who also have genuine seizures.

- *Fictitious epilepsy*: remember that this is not uncommon. Obtain the name of someone other than the parent who has witnessed an attack and who can be contacted; for example, school teacher.

Notes

- Children who are suspected or known to have seizures need complete physical examination.

- If the child is asked to count to 100, hesitations may reveal brief absence seizures.

- Starting anticonvulsants is a serious decision. If there is still doubt whether the child has seizures after taking a detailed history, consider asking the child to hyperventilate for 3 minutes. In susceptible children this procedure will induce generalized absence seizures in most, and complex partial seizures in a proportion. If a good history of generalized convulsive seizures has been obtained there is no point performing this test. **NB** *In view of the potential danger, this procedure should be carried out only under careful supervision including the availability of drugs and equipment for the management of status epilepticus.*

Epilepsy in adults

The history

Ask the patient if have they recently had a blackout and when exactly?

Obtain a description of the attack. This should include a description by the patient complemented by a description from an informant who has witnessed an attack. The patient may have had more than one form of attack. Ask both patient and informant to describe a typical attack from the beginning.

Pre-ictal

Can the patient (or close observer) predict when an attack will happen minutes/hours before it does? How? — change in mood (irritability, dysphoria); cognition (inattentiveness, confused behaviour); build-up of minor seizures, (absences, myoclonic jerks).

Do these features resolve once the attack has occurred?

The epileptic attack

The presence of aura indicates focal cortical onset and strongly suggests underlying brain damage or disease. Is there any immediate warning of the attack or does the patient lose consciousness abruptly? If there is a warning, how long does it last? Does it last long enough to take avoiding action? Auras rarely exceed one minute in duration. Enquire after the aura content. Alimentary (epigastric sensations) and psychic (*déjà vu*, hallucinatory) auras suggest a temporal lobe focus. A sensory–motor 'march' suggests a primary sensory–motor cortical focus.

- Is consciousness lost suddenly or gradually?
- Is the patient completely unconscious or do they retain some awareness of what is going on around them? (if so, what?)

What were they told of how they were while unconscious? Do they fall or slump to the ground or are they able to maintain their posture? Are they perfectly still or do they make movements? If the latter, are the movements rhythmic or irregular? Which parts of the body are involved? Are they more marked on one side of the body than the other? Is there any spread or are they generalized from the beginning? Is there any initial rotation of the head/eyes to one side?

- How long does this phase last?

  If the patient retains posture:

- Do they carry out any automatism (co-ordinated movement — fumbling, searching, etc.)?
- Are there any tongue/lip/cheek biting episodes or urinary incontinence?

  After the patient appears to regain consciousness, how are they:

- Confused, sleepy, delayed speech recovery, quick recovery?

  Are any other epileptic episodes described:

- Absences, myoclonic jerks?

Course

When was the first seizure? When was the patient first investigated? What was the patient/family told? When were anticonvulsants first started? Enquire about past and present seizure frequency.

- *Seizure pattern*: diurnal — nocturnal (how is this recognized) — both
- *Precipitating factors*: stress — menses — photic stimulation (self-induced flicker effect, TV, nightclub stroboscope) — lack of sleep — non-compliance with medication
- *Predisposing factors*: family history of epilepsy — difficult birth — febrile fits during infancy — history of head injury, brain infection (meningitis, encephalitis) — seizures following immunization.

Diagnostic features to look out for

Other diagnostic possibilities

- *Pseudo-seizures*: atypical features to the seizure — opisthotonos, pelvic thrusting, thrashing limbs, resists examination.
- *Panic disorder*: preceded by hyperventilation, chest discomfort, peripheral paraesthesiae, carpopedal spasm.
- *Alcohol related*: history of excessive alcohol consumption — seizures occur during drinking bouts or immediately after withdrawal.
- *Others*: cardiac syncope, vasovagal episodes.

Differential diagnosis of confused behaviours occurring in the context of epilepsy

- *Post-ictal psychosis*: follows exacerbation of seizure activity, post-ictal latent period of normality before psychotic symptoms begin, clinical picture dominated by confusion, hallucinations, and affective disturbance (twilight state), history of previous episodes, usually lasts only a few days and is self-limiting.
- *Post-ictal confusion*: history of recent seizure, patient confused and drowsy, usually resolves within a couple of hours.

- *Alcohol intoxication*: evident signs of drunken behaviour, alcohol on breath, known history.

- *Head injury*: careful neurological examination indicated if recent history of head injury or evidence of scalp/facial injuries.

- *Anticonvulsant medication*: complaints of drowsiness, poor co-ordination. On examination nystagmus, dysarthria, and ataxia. There may be a history of recent change in drug dosage.

Immediate management

Related to epilepsy

- If seizures are *well controlled*. Find out from patient who/where epilepsy is treated and copy clinical correspondence with details of psychiatric diagnosis and treatment.

- If seizures are *poorly controlled*. Obtain details of medication, check compliance, request plasma anticonvulsant levels, and, once available, correspond as above.

- The patient is *confused and disoriented*. This will usually be due to post-ictal confusion, but see differential diagnosis of confused behaviours above. Post-ictal confusion will rarely exceed 6 hours. Observe until recovered, otherwise admit.

- *A seizure occurs*. Most minor seizures are very brief and do not require any intervention. If it is a major tonic–clonic seizure, ensure airway (turn patient on side and remove false teeth) and guard patient from hard edge/cornered objects that could be injurious. Do not restrain or attempt to separate teeth. Give clonazepam, 1 mg IV or Diazemuls 10 mg IV. If seizure is prolonged (more than 5 minutes) or status (repeated seizures without intervening recovery of consciousness) develops, repeat injection and request immediate medical assistance. *Prolonged seizure activity/status is a medical emergency and may lead to hypoxia, hypotension, and hyperthermia and may result in permanent brain damage.*

Related to psychiatric illness

In general, immediate management is the same as it would be for the psychiatric condition were epilepsy absent. However, there are exceptions:

- *Acute psychotic illness*: this, in a patient not known to be psychotic is usually post-ictal. Unless relatives are used to dealing with such episodes, it is best to admit.

- *Pseudo-seizures*: the clinician may suspect, and even observe a seizure that appears to be non-epileptic. It is better to pass these observations on to the GP/specialist who usually treats a patient's epilepsy rather than comment directly. If in doubt treat as for epilepsy.

Response to treatment

Commonly prescribed anticonvulsant drugs

- *Carbamazepine, phenytoin, phenobarbitone, and primidone* are first-choice anticonvulsants against most seizure types with the exception of general absence seizures (petit mal). The last two drugs are now rarely prescribed because of their potential as drugs of abuse.

- *Lamotrigine*, a more recent drug, is effective against a wide range of seizure types including generalized absence seizures.

- *Sodium valproate* is a first choice in primary generalized epilepsy, less so in partial epilepsy.

- *Ethosuximide* is a first-choice drug against generalized absence seizures.

- *Clonazepam* is a first-choice drug against myoclonic and atypical generalized absence seizures.

- *Clobazam, gabapentin, and vigabatrin* are second-choice anticonvulsants against partial and secondary generalized seizures.

Careful monitoring of anticonvulsant blood levels is essential, especially at times of change in drug regime.

Some patients with intractable epilepsy may be eligible for brain surgery.

Course

In most patients (approximately 80 per cent) seizures will be effectively controlled by the first anticonvulsant prescribed. In patients with additional neurological and neuropsychiatric disabilities, control may not be so readily achieved and polytherapy may be unavoidable. Partial seizures are more difficult to control than primary generalized ones.

Generalized absence seizures usually resolve by the third decade.

Seizures developing for the first time in mid- or late life may be associated with progressive underlying pathology and should be investigated with particular care.

Investigations

The investigation of newly suspected epileptic seizures include an electroencephalogram (EEG), and, particularly in the case of partial seizures, a search for a primary cause. This would include brain imaging (computed tomography, CT; magnetic resonance imaging, MRI) and routine haematological and biochemical tests. A waking scalp EEG will only show relevant abnormalities in about 50 per cent of cases: a sleep EEG is often more informative. In the case of epilepsy of late onset, periodic re-scanning may be desirable.

When, on clinical grounds, there is considerable doubt about the epileptic nature of the seizures and a routine EEG remains negative, a prolonged EEG (telemetry)/video recording may capture a seizure and confirm or refute the diagnosis. In most centres this investigation is carried out over a 5-day period whilst the patient is in hospital. Seizures must occur with sufficient frequency for this to be an effective investigation.

Patients considered for surgery may undergo tests that assist in localization. These may include telemetry with special electrode placement (foramen ovale, subdural, intracerebral), specialized MRI procedures (volumetric hippocampal measurements, proton spectroscopy), detailed neuropsychological assessment, carotid amytal measurements to determine cerebral dominance and lateralization of memory function, and measures of cerebral blood flow (single photon emission computed tomography, SPECT; positron emission tomography, PET) to identify any filling defect.

The mute or inaccessible patient

Definitions

Mutism is the inability or unwillingness to speak, resulting in the absence or marked paucity of verbal output. It may be isolated, but often occurs clustered with other disturbances of behaviour, level of consciousness, affect, motor disturbance, or thought processes and may be due to an organic or non-organic disorder.

Stupor is a term used by neurologists as a stage on the continuum with comatose, implying reduced consciousness, but in common psychiatric terminology it constitutes preserved awareness with severe psychomotor inhibition. Mutism is invariably present in stupor. In general, these terms should not be used in isolation, but should be combined with a detailed description of the clinical features.

History

The history will need to be obtained from informants — relatives, keyworkers, neighbours, etc. In particular, the following should be established: How long has the patient been mute? Was the development sudden or gradual? Was there a stressful precipitant, or did the patient seem overly sad or happy in the prodrome? Is the mutism partial or complete? Is it specific to one situation, e.g. school? Does any of the patient's behaviour seem odd or bizarre? How does the patient function in day-to-day life — eating, drinking, sleeping, continence, social activities, etc.? Is there a past history of psychiatric disorder, conversion disorder, neurological or medical illness? What drugs have been prescribed/taken?

Examination

A general examination of physical state — temperature, pulse, blood pressure, and state of hydration (look at the tongue) should be undertaken. The presence of mutism also demands a full neurological examination, beginning with an assessment of the level of consciousness. An impaired level of consciousness, or the presence of focal neurological signs should lead to prompt referral to a physician or neurologist.

In particular, investigate whether the patient can articulate (by making lip movements or whispering), phonate (by humming or coughing). Take note of the eye movements, is the patient watchful, making purposive movements implying awareness of surroundings (Beware 'roving eyes' in the unconscious patient)? Are the eyes deviated to one side or another (eyes deviate away from a focal lesion, but towards an epileptiform focus during a seizure)? Does the patient with closed eyes resist opening? Is reclosure of the eyes slow and uniform, as occurs in the unconscious patients (this can not be simulated) or is there resistance?

Is communication possible by other means; for example, writing/signing? Are there any attempts to speak? To what extent is comprehension affected? (Pure motor (Broca's) dysphasia is normally accompanied by frustrated attempts at communication and comprehension is relatively intact.) Speech delay is evident in a substantial minority of children with elective mutism.

In the mental state examination, note the state of mental arousal and motor activity, is there associated motor retardation? What is indicated by facial expression, does he/she appear elated, anxious, frightened, sad, or angry? Describe any grimaces, gestures, or mannerisms. Is there any evidence of attempts at communication, or does the patient seem unconcerned by his/her state, for example is there '*belle indifference*'? Does he/she appear to be preoccupied, perhaps by hallucinations, ruminations, or paranoia?

Differential diagnosis of mutism

Psychiatric disorders

- *Psychotic disorder*: mutism may occur as a response to a delusional system in schizophrenia or as part of the negative symptoms in association with reduced drive.

- *Affective disorder*: mutism in depression may result in psychomotor retardation or nihilism, whereas in mania, it may occur as part of a manic stupor.

- *Elective mutism*: this is most often seen in children, where there is emotionally determined selectivity in speaking, it is associated with social anxiety, withdrawal, or sensitivity.

- *Pervasive developmental disorders*: the use of language is delayed and often idiosyncratic, although mutism is rare. It is accompanied by impairments in social interaction, and in a restricted range of interests.

- *Obsessional slowness*: this may be accompanied by severely restricted speech output.

- *Somatoform /dissociative disorder*: in psychogenic dysphonia, the ability to phonate may help in differentiating it from an organic condition. Post-traumatic stress disorder may also be accompanied by mutism.

- *Factitious disorder:* this is rare, but may occur in situations where divulgence of information may be detrimental; for example, with a pending court case.

Neurological disorders

- *Lesions of cortex*: (for example, frontal, speech areas), brain-stem (for example, akinetic mutism [coma vigil] — 'locked in syndrome'), basal ganglia (such as Parkinson's disease, Wilson's disease).

- *Infective*: for example, herpes encephalitis, HIV related disease.

- *Drugs*: for example, neuroleptics (which may cause dystonic reactions involving the tongue and jaw muscles, as well as torti-collis, laryngeal spasm, and occulogyric crises), lithium, seda-tives, antiepileptics.

- *Seizure related*: for example, during or after complex partial seizures, absence attacks, partial status.

- *Deafness*: which may give rise to speech delay in children and impaired production of speech.

Investigations

These should include haematology, biochemistry including blood sugar, toxin/drug screen, syphilis serology, endocrine screen, chest

X-ray (CXR), EEG (which may indicate localized epileptiform activity, although its absence does not necessarily exclude seizures), and brain imaging with CT or MRI.

Initial treatment

Once serious neurological disorder has been excluded, a period of observation is often valuable. However, the presence of severe psychomotor retardation in depressive disorder or manic stupor may require urgent treatment and electroconvulsive therapy (ECT) should be considered. Treatment of dystonic reactions should be initiated quickly as this is frightening and painful for patients. Intravenous or intramuscular procyclidine is spectacularly effective.

The catatonic patient

Definitions

Catatonia is a term which was originally associated with a variety of psychiatric illnesses, and later specifically with schizophrenia. It is currently recognized as a non-specific syndrome, which occurs in a variety of organic states as well as in psychotic, affective, and somatoform psychiatric disorders. Catatonia is characterized by abnormal motor behaviour, with periods of hyper- and hypo-activity. Mutism and stupor are common, and it is often associated with features such as posturing, waxy flexibility, negativism, impulsiveness, stereotypies, mannerisms, command automatisms, echopraxia, or echolalia.

History

The ability of the catatonic patient to give a history may be preserved, and history-taking should then proceed along normal lines. More commonly, however, communication is impaired, and assessment must be undertaken as for the mute patient, questioning relevant informants. If communication is possible, the patient should be asked about any meaning attached to the postures adopted, which may lead to the uncovering of a delusional system, the degree to which the patient is distressed by the motor symptoms (it is important to distinguish from the mental and physical agitation of neuroleptic-induced akathisia), and whether passive movement is painful (which is often the case in waxy flexibility). Also ask about previous episodes of catatonia, as well as past psychiatric history.

Examination

As with mutism, the presence of catatonia demands a full physical examination. Patients may shift rapidly into a period of catatonic overactivity, which could render people close by to physical danger, therefore vigilance should be retained during examination. The catatonic patient is at risk of dehydration, rhabdomyolysis, sepsis, venous thrombosis, and pressure sores; examination should pay particular attention to these factors, as well as excluding the organic causes of catatonia. The following phenomena should be elicited where possible:

- *Automatic obedience*: the patient gives a robot-like response to any instruction, however silly.
- *Negativism*: a similarly stereotyped response, but the opposite of what was requested.
- *Waxy flexibility*: the patient's limbs can be moved slowly into a new posture passively, but return gradually to the previously sustained posture
- *'Psychological pillow'*: on lying down, the patient's head remains held a few inches above the bed.
- *Ambitendence*: the patient begins to make a movement, but before completing it, begins to make the opposite movement.
- *Echolalia*: the patient repeats the examiner's words or phrases.
- *Echopraxia*: the patient repeats any movements made by the examiner.
- *Mannerisms*: the patient exhibits repetitive goal-directed behaviours.

- *Stereotypies*: the patient exhibits repetitive non-goal-directed behaviours.

Differential diagnosis

Psychiatric disorders

- *Affective disorder*: depression is probably the commonest psychiatric cause of catatonia and is considerably more common than mania. It often develops slowly; therefore, history may be particularly informative.

- *Schizophrenic disorder*: 'catatonic schizophrenia' is relatively rare now in western practice, although catatonic motor disorders (namely, a part of the catatonic syndrome) are commonly seen in all subgroups of schizophrenia. Catatonia is a relatively common presentation of puerperal psychosis.

- *Obsessional slowness*: catatonic features may be due to severe obsessive compulsive disorders (OCD). Access to the typical mental state (with ruminations and obsessions) may be available from observation or from the informant's history.

- *Somatoform/dissociative*: this is rare and requires both the absence of physical or functional psychiatric aetiology, as well as positive evidence of psychogenic causation.

Neurological disorders

- *Lesions of cortex*: (frontal and temporal lobes), brainstem, basal ganglia, limbic system, or diencephalon [for example, tumour, cerebral thrombosis or haemorrhage, head injury, infective (including encephalitis lethargica and syphilis)].

- *Drugs*: for example, neuroleptics (neuroleptic malignant syndrome — catatonia with rigidity, and temperature and autonomic instability) (see p. 181), lithium, morphine derivatives.

- *Toxins*: for example, carbon monoxide poisoning, alcohol damage, ecstasy, alcohol.

- *Seizure related*: for example, simple partial or complex partial seizures.

- *Systemic*: for example, renal, hepatic failure, endocrine disorder, connective tissue disorders (particularly cerebral SLE).
- *Other*: for example, acute intermittent or coproporphyria, vitamin deficiency.

In addition, there are a proportion of patients who present with recurrent catatonia in whom no psychiatric or neurological disorder can be found. This subgroup seems to be familial, and spontaneous recovery is the general rule.

Investigations

This should include haematology, biochemistry including blood sugar, toxin/drug screen, syphilis serology, endocrine screen, CXR, EEG (which may indicate localized epileptiform activity, although its absence does not necessarily exclude seizures), and brain imaging with CT or MRI. In the case of diagnostic difficulty, abreaction may reverse the catatonia of the functional psychoses for a short time, allowing the emergence of 'hidden' psychopathology; the response to a single ECT may also be useful diagnostically.

Initial treatment

Supportive treatment, including fluid and electrolyte replacement, antibiotics, and anticoagulation should be initiated where indicated. Once treatable neurological causes have been excluded, consideration should be given to the early or even emergency use of ECT, since patients are at risk of a number of physical complications. Benzodiazepines, intravenously and then orally, have been shown to be of value acutely whilst neuroleptics begin to take effect. Neuroleptic malignant syndrome should be considered a medical emergency, and advice should be sought urgently. Initial treatment is discontinuation of the neuroleptic, supportive treatment of autonomic and temperature regulation failure, and treatment with dantrolene, benzodiazepines, and dopamine agonists.

6
Summary, formulation, progress notes

The summary

This is an important document which should be drawn up with care. Its purpose is to provide a concise description of all the important aspects of the case, enabling others who are unfamiliar with the patient to grasp the essential features of the problem without needing to search elsewhere for further information.

The first part should be completed within a week of admission and be drawn up for typing under the following headings:

- Reason for referral
- Present illness
- Personal history
  - Family history
  - Personal history
  - Childhood
  - Occupations
  - Marriage and children
  - Previous personality
  - Physical illness
  - Previous mental illness
- Physical examination
- Mental state.

The summary should cover all important aspects of the mental state, and be drawn up under whichever of the subheadings in the main schema are necessary to achieve this. The six subheadings of personal history listed above should always be included, and others from the main schema introduced as appropriate.

The second part should be completed within 1 week of discharge and be laid out under the following headings:

- Investigations
- Treatment and progress.
- Final diagnosis (or diagnoses) together with the diagnostic code number from the International Classification of Diseases (ICD-10 number: see p. 281).
- Prognosis (make a predictive statement related to symptoms and social adaptation, rather than terms like guarded, good, or poor).
- Condition on discharge.
- Care plan (see p. 230).

The completed summary should be short enough to cover about two sides of A4 paper when typed.

The summary of a readmission should include the full range of categories listed here, unless the last admission was very recent and it has been established that no significant change has occurred in the family history and personal history in the interim.

References to highly confidential matters (criminal acts, sexual revelations, etc.) should be included only if their omission would produce a serious distortion of the overall picture. Often it will be preferable to include only a veiled reference followed by 'see notes' in brackets. The summary should identify which professional workers are to be responsible for different aspects of the patient's care in the future.

Components of pattern recognition

A summary is a **descriptive** account of collected data: **objective** and impartial. In contrast, a formulation is a clinical opinion: weighing up the pros and cons of conflicting evidence, that leads to a diagnostic choice. An opinion inevitably implies a **subjective** viewpoint, by virtue of assigning relative importance to each piece of evidence; in doing so, both theoretical bias and past personal experiences invariably come into play. No matter how accurate the final verdict, an analysis is inextricably bound up with subjective judgements and decisions. When assessing the same patient, two experts may produce two similar summaries, but two different formulations with divergent conclusions. This is the fundamental difference: a summary is descriptive, whereas a formulation is analytical. Therefore, a summary calls for the qualities of thoroughness, restraint, and objectivity; while a formulation demands the composite skill of methodical thinking, incisive analysis, and intelligent presentation.

Formulating a case with clarity and precision is probably the most testing yet challenging and crucial part of a psychiatric assessment. The skill of writing a good formulation depends upon the ability to differentiate what are merely the incidental and circumstantial biographical details from what are the salient and discriminatory features and it is this that forms the cornerstone of a clinical diagnosis. Certain features are discriminatory because they support one diagnosis as the more likely candidate and discount another diagnosis as less likely. Extracting these relevant features to construct meaningful patterns is the skill often called **pattern recognition**.

Gathering information about a patient — as in taking a history or performing a physical and mental state examination — is not carried out in a passive and routine way. It is an active hypothesis-testing process, in which the clinician starts out with a number of possible hypotheses about the nature of a patient's illness and then proceeds to verify and falsify each one until he arrives at the few final most plausible causes.

There are two components to the process of 'pattern recognition': first, identifying a number of key features that form a familiar constellation — **gestalt recognition**; this is how you recognize that a large grey animal with a long trunk and big ears is an elephant. If you have seen an elephant before, you can instantly recognize one and can readily distinguish it from a pig or an orang-utan. The second differentiates two similar patterns by eliciting the most discriminating features — **pattern differentiation**. This allows you to identify the species of the elephant, provided that you have specialist knowledge about all the species of elephants and about the specific features that characterize each species.

There are four main reasons why a piece of information is discriminatory.

First, it can be one of several *cardinal features that constitute a syndrome*. In the classification of disorders, clinical syndromes can be grouped into monothetic syndromes or polythetic syndromes. In a monothetic syndrome, it its necessary for all syndrome-defining features to be present, for example to make the diagnosis of hyperkinetic disorder, the triad of hyperactivity, inattentiveness, and impulsivity needs to be present. These features are highly discriminatory and their absence excludes the diagnosis.

In Asperger's syndrome (which is often mistaken for paranoid or schizoid personality disorder) if aloofness and social impairment occur together with odd speech patterns, perseverating routines, circumscribed interests, often bizarre hobbies (such as obsessively collecting photographs of aerials or pylons) — then Asperger's syndrome is the more likely diagnosis. The addition of one or two of these syndrome-defining features completely alters the weighting of the differential diagnosis, because now the symptoms of aloofness and social impairment become the composite parts of the Asperger's constellation. Other examples are Cotard's syndrome, Capgras syndrome, Tourette's syndrome, and Ganser's syndrome; each one has a specific constellation of symptoms and signs that characterize the syndrome.

Second, it can be a *pathognomonic feature of a disorder* since it is unique to a disorder, rarely occurring elsewhere. Although helpful when present, its absence does not exclude the disorder. In a polythetic syndrome, only some of the syndrome-defining features need to be present. Edward's seven features of alcohol-dependence syndrome can serve as an example: compulsion, stereotyped repertoire, primacy, tolerance, withdrawal, reinstatement, and eye opener. All of them are highly specific to an alcohol-dependent drinker, rarely found in control drinkers or other disorders, but not all need to be present simultaneously. Delirium is another example, characterized by impairment of consciousness (as other features of the condition are widely variable). Other variable features roughly fall into two common patterns: in the first, the patient is restless and over-reacting to stimuli, exhibiting psychotic symptoms; in the second, he is lethargic and quiet with few psychotic symptoms. Impairment of consciousness reliably distinguishes delirium from other conditions, while the two subtypes of delirium are recognized by pattern differentiation.

Third, it can be *one of a set* of diagnostic criteria — as stipulated by ICD-10 or DSMIV — and its presence arbitrarily defines a disorder. Schizophrenia and depression are both examples of this kind of syndrome: there is no single pathognomonic symptom that has to be present. One of these conditions is said to be present when more than a critical number of typical symptoms are present. The distinction between sickness and health is arbitrary.

Fourth, it can be the *sign that distinguishes two otherwise identical conditions*, although such a feature may be neither pathognomonic nor defining of a disorder when considered in isolation. Both conditions share many common clinical features, except some small specific hallmarks — like differentiating a pair of identical twins: if you know one has a little mole over the left eye and the other one has a small scar on the right thumb, you can distinguish the two at a glance. This is the skill of 'pattern differentiation'. The differentiating hallmarks may not be pathognomonic features because they may not characterize the condition when considered in isolation: they are important only as the features peculiar to one twin or another.

For example, an apparent generalized intellectual impairment ('pseudo-dementia') can be difficult to differentiate from that caused by dementia in the elderly. A useful distinguishing sign is that the depressed patients are often reluctant to answer questions and give 'don't know' answers. In contrast to this, the patients with true dementia are willing to ramble on in response to any questions asked. Therefore, it is vitally important to elicit these signs because their presence is helpful in differentiating the two conditions. In a demented patient, the presence of prominent extrapyramidal symptoms, visual hallucinations, and hypersensitivity to neuroleptics would 'recruit' all dementia features to the diagnosis of Lewy body dementia.

The formulation

A diagnosis involves a **nomothetic** (literally 'law-giving') process. This means that all cases included within the identified category have one or more properties in common. By contrast, the formulation is an **idiographic** process (literally 'picture of the individual'). This means that it includes the unique characteristics of each patient's case which are needed for the process of management. So, while nomothetic processes are the only way we can advance knowledge about diseases, we use idiographic methods to understand and study the individual.

The format of the formulation

The formulation follows a logical sequence.

Demographic data

Begin with the name, age, occupation, and marital status of the patient.

Descriptive formulation

Describe the nature of onset — for example, acute or insidious; the total duration of the present illness; and the course; for instance, cyclic or deteriorating. Then list the main phenomena (namely, symptoms and signs) that characterize the disorder. As you become more experienced you should try to be selective by featuring those phenomena that are most important, either because of their greater diagnostic specificity or because of their predominance in severity or duration. Avoid long lists of minor or transient symptoms and negative findings. These basic data are chiefly derived from the history of the present illness, the mental state, and physical examinations and are used to determine the syndrome diagnosis in the next section. Note that this is not usually the place to bring in other aspects of the history: that comes later. If we know the diagnosis of a previous episode of mental illness, this should also be taken into account, but remember, the present disorder may not be connected and the diagnosis may be different.

Differential diagnosis

List, in order of probability, all diagnoses that should be considered and include any disorders that you will wish to investigate. These will usually be syndrome diagnoses based on the descriptive formulation above. Give the evidence for and against each diagnosis that you consider. Include any current physical illness which may account for some or all of the phenomena. A common error is to include, for example, thyroid function studies in the investigations without including thyroid disease in the differential diagnosis. If you think a condition is worth investigating then you are obviously including it in your differential diagnosis; if it's not worth mentioning don't bother to investigate it.

Remember that in addition to the primary diagnosis you may need to consider a supplementary diagnosis; for example, alcoholism in a patient presenting with delirium, or a personality disorder in a patient with an anxiety state.

Aetiology

The various factors that have contributed should be evident mainly from the family and personal histories, the history of previous illness, and the premorbid personality. Try to answer two questions: why has this patient developed this particular disorder, and why has the disorder developed at this particular time?

Investigations

List all investigations that are required to support your preferred diagnosis and to rule out the alternatives, and also any that you think are required to improve your understanding of the aetiology. Give reasons for the investigations if they are not self-evident. Include all sources of additional information.

Treatment

Outline the treatment plan that you wish to follow. This should stem logically from your discussion of the aetiology as well as from the diagnosis.

Prognosis

Describe the expected outcome of management of this illness episode, both with regard to the symptoms and also subsequent function; for example, self-care and return to the community. Consider the risk of subsequent relapse.

Progress notes

Regular progress notes, *signed and dated*, are a vital part of every case record. They should describe the treatment the patient is receiving (with dates of starting and finishing, and dosages of all drugs), significant changes in mental state, and any important events involving the patient. They should also record the opinions expressed by consultants at ward rounds and case conferences. Although these notes must be detailed enough to convey an accurate picture of the patient's treatment and his response to it, they should not normally contain lengthy verbatim accounts of conversations between patient and doctor. Notes which are excessively long are never read.

Handover notes

A *handover note* should be written whenever the patient is transferred from the care of one junior doctor to another, summarizing the salient features and outlining future plans. This is particularly important in the case of out-patients for whom there is no formal summary or formulation.

7
Special interview situations

The patient who demands proof that you care

Some very lonely people rely on their doctors and other professional attendants for social contact. Many of these accept the limitations and boundaries of the professional relationship and 'play the game' by generating the kinds of problems they know you deal with — side-effects of medication, new somatic complaints, etc. A small number make escalating demands based on the assertion that you don t really care — it is only a professional relationship to you. In order to demonstrate that you do care, you may find yourself putting them at the end of an out-patient clinic so that you can spend longer with them than with other patients. Then you may find that everyone else has gone home by the time you finish the consultation. As you recognize the person's really desperate state you may encourage them to phone you between appointments. Then as it is clear that once-weekly visits to the clinic are insufficient you find yourself offering extra appointments outside working hours. By this time you have a Very Special Patient, although often none of your tokens of care are having the desired effect. Far from the patient becoming happier and more able to face independent life, you are now apparently indispensable to the patient's very survival. Indeed, suicide threats and gestures may be used to ensure you remain centrally involved in their care. Frightened childlike behaviour may elicit an impulse to comfort the patient — holding hands, an arm round their shoulder. DON'T, you are in danger!

It is not that such people are not desperate and lonely and have not suffered terrible deprivation and cruelty in childhood; it is only that you will never be able to prove you care enough, not even if you were to adopt them into your own family. (Incredibly such things do happen.) The danger for you is that a central motivation in becoming a doctor — the relief of suffering and the wish to heal damaged minds and bodies is being abused and your professional identity is under threat. Sexual contact between doctor and patient is far from uncommon and may happen as the result of a series of short steps, starting as outlined above. The contact can be heterosexual or homosexual, and it is an unequivocal breech of professional ethics.

The cardinal rule in caring for patients who demand proof that you care is not to become isolated with them. The first step is to seek supervision from senior colleagues and the second is to arrive at a care plan involving the multidisciplinary team. Continuing psychodynamic supervision of such cases is essential to optimize care and to protect the carers.

The patient who solicits erotic involvement

From time-to-time a patient may develop an erotic attachment to the doctor and declare undying passion. Sometimes this can be managed by simply explaining that it is impossible for you to continue as the doctor if the patient insists on treating you as a potential lover. Indeed this may be the unconscious motivation of the patient's attraction, so that one could pose the question: 'What is it about my being your doctor that you wish to avoid?'.

If the patient persists importunately there is no alternative but to transfer his care to a colleague, explaining that further contact between you and the patient will henceforth cease. Further harassment and stalking are matters for the forensic psychiatrist and possibly the police.

When such cases do arise it is important to examine one's own dress and behaviour to ensure that you are not unconsciously signalling availability or even behaving seductively towards the patient. A good rule of thumb is to seek supervision of such cases from a senior colleague or possibly a psychotherapist.

The patient who brings gifts

In psychiatry one can expect expressions of gratitude less often than in other specialities. There is no problem with a parting gift at the end of a course of treatment — accept it graciously, unless it be cash. The patient who brings gifts during treatment is more of a problem. Assume the gift contains a hidden message and find a way of addressing it without being churlish: for example, examples of work the patient has done (pottery in occupational therapy, a knitted teacosy, a cake, a published article) may be important signs of competence and recovery; they may also be a concrete token of the patient's wish to remain in your mind and be part of your non-professional life. This is not a sin, but is better put into words than left unspoken.

Ever more extravagant and inappropriate gifts suggest the patient has privately elevated you to a demi-god, to be placated, propitiated, and perhaps expecting one day untold benefits in return. This is a more direct attack on the professional relationship and needs to be addressed: 'I really cannot accept such an expensive gift, I wonder if you fear I will not take you seriously if you come empty-handed', or some variation on this.

The patient who is disinhibited

At its most harmless, disinhibition may take the form of making personal remarks, cracking tactless jokes, and asking intrusive personal questions to the doctor. Do not rise to personal remarks, fail to laugh at tactless jokes, and fend off personal questions. In general, respond in a muted and subdued way rather than returning the affective tone of the patient.

More difficult to deal with is the patient who enters one's personal space, either to touch, stroke, or hit the doctor. The former should also be fended off, perhaps distracting the patient by reminding them what you wanted them to do: 'You were telling me about the voices that you hear'. The latter is more difficult to deal with, and you may have to withdraw and try again later, or return accompanied by a nurse. It is especially important to do this if the doctor is examining a sexually disinhibited patient of the opposite gender — it is in the doctor's own interests.

The patient who refuses to leave

Stand at the end of the consultation to signal firmly that it is over. Say: 'I am afraid I am going to have to ask you to leave'.

Appeal to the person s better nature: 'If you don t go now I will be keeping others waiting' (this, of course, may be the reason the patient will not leave). Finally: 'I am going to call for someone to escort you out of my room', and telephone for help. This is preferable to any attempt to coax or manhandle the patient on your own.

Managing awkward situations

BE PREPARED: expect the unexpected — many awkward situations arise because the doctor has been only half awake to the fact that psychiatric patients, at least from time-to-time, do not behave reasonably.

If you are called out of hours to see a patient you do not know on a ward or in accident and emergency, as far as possible inform yourself about the patient before seeing him. Read the medical and nursing notes, especially the Part I Summary, Formulations, Care plans and reports of management and ward round decisions. Ask to be briefed by the senior nurse on duty or by the accompanying friend or relative of the patient in casualty. Where possible ask the nurse to be present while you interview the patient and *never* conduct a physical examination alone. If, for any reason, you decide to interview the patient on your own, first of all be clear how to call for help.

Position yourself within reach of the telephone, know the number to call for help. Be sure there is somebody within earshot who knows to respond quickly to raised voices or furniture being violently relocated. If there is a 'panic button', stay within reach of it. If the patient wishes to leave, allow him to do so, and do not obstruct his path to the door. However, it is generally safer to be sitting near to the door yourself. If the patient produces a weapon, terminate the interview as quickly as possible by explaining to the patient that it is impossible for you to help him when he is armed, but that you will be pleased to continue to talk to him as soon as he has given his weapon to someone to look after for him. Leave as soon as you have said this, if the patient will allow you to do so: offer to fetch him a cup of tea or coffee while he thinks about what you have said. If the patient will not allow you to leave stay calm, and chat to the patient about neutral matters; if you can press the panic button without increasing the risk to yourself do so.

The patient who demands drugs

Often the story given is one of a lost prescription or of a sudden motivation to stop illicit drug use. There are no rules about how to deal with this situation, but the following points may help:

- Take a good history of exactly which drugs and how much the patient is consuming.
- If they do claim to have lost a prescription who was it prescribed by? Can you check with them? Where is it being dispensed? Pharmacists keep good records and will often be open late.
- Do not prescribe unless you feel confident you are doing so safely.
- Never start a prescription that cannot be continued safely; for example, by a local addiction service.
- Remember opiate withdrawal is not physically dangerous, but benzodiazepine withdrawal and alcohol withdrawal can be.
- The patient has probably been using illicit drugs for a long time. They can continue for another day or two until an appropriate referral is made.
- Try to consult a specialist.

The patient who threatens violence

Even the most skilful clinician will occasionally be faced with a patient whose behaviour escalates such that physical assault seems imminent, or who even offers violence in so many words (but see Chapter 1, pp. 12–14). Usually, this arises when some real or perceived threat to his physical or psychological integrity has made the patient both very frightened and very angry — essentially, he feels that things are getting out of his control.

Particularly high-risk situations include interviewing patients whose delusional beliefs are that harm is imminent, or telling a patient of a clinical decision to detain or treat him against his will. Patients who are disinhibited by drugs or alcohol are especially prone to sudden aggression.

Much can be done to defuse a crisis before violence erupts, and not just for your own benefit: other staff will avoid the risks of coming to your aid, and the patient will escape adverse labelling and possibly even a criminal conviction. Anticipate your interview with an unknown, possibly disturbed patient as follows:

- Read the records for information about the patient's likely mental state and any previous history of violence and substance misuse.

- Ask the nursing staff about the patient's current behaviour, concerns and whether they think he has been drinking. Junior nursing staff will often defer to you on the question as to whether the patient is safe to interview alone (even if you know far less about him than they) unless you make it clear that you value their views.

- Arrange to use an interview room that can be easily observed by staff who know where you are, or who are prepared to wait outside if necessary. The room should ideally have an alarm button that is close to hand; never allow the patient to sit between you and the door, which should be easily opened from the inside.

- On the other hand, the room should also allow for a degree of privacy and quiet.

The interview itself should be conducted in a polite and, if anything, slightly formal manner: not only will this promote a psychological distance between you that discourages violence, but by treating the patient as someone important, you will increase his self-esteem. Do not invade his personal space, touch him, tower over him, or sit behind a large desk, but rather make an effort to build up rapport. Tell the patient who you are and that you want to do your best to help him. Take time to listen to his concerns, and if they are delusional, acknowledge his fear, distress, or anger rather than arguing about their veracity. It often helps to tell the patient that they are frightening everyone, as they may genuinely be unaware of this. Similarly, asking a female relative or member of staff to sit in with you may help to modify his behaviour.

With some patients these techniques will fail, especially if they have been drinking, have very fixed beliefs, or are very aroused. If your intuition tells you to beware, listen to it. If you are clearly getting nowhere, do not increase the patient's frustration by prolonging the interview unnecessarily. Usually, the matter can only be resolved by telling the patient that you want him to do something, such as stay in hospital, take medication, or go into the seclusion room. By now, you will know that this is going to be provocative, and if you are alone with him it will usually be best to leave the room and fetch help — if necessary, tell the patient that you are going to consult a senior colleague. Confronting such a patient with medication should only be done with a control and restraint team in the room with you, and the medication prepared and ready to be administered.

The assessment of dangerousness

Recently, the general approach to the problem of 'dangerousness' has altered. The central focus has shifted from the question of whether a particular patient is or is not 'dangerous' to an assessment of the risk he poses in a particular situation under specific circumstances. This paradigm shift has facilitated clearer thinking about patients potential dangerous behaviour in that it highlights the importance of psychiatric decision taking, the information on which decisions are based, and their underlying logic.

Theoretical framework

Recognize that some level of risk is present

Just as the psychiatrist will automatically consider the likelihood of his or her patient committing suicide, so thinking about whether the patient may harm others must become routine. As with suicide, sometimes the risk of violence is unmistakable. However, on other occasions it may be much less so. While apparently obvious, it needs to be stressed that recognition that the risk exists is the essential first step in the assessment of the likelihood of self-harm and violence to others.

In the case of suicide, actuarial data have helped raise the question of risk in an individual by pointing to their membership of a vulnerable group. Similarly, the possibility of violent behaviour may be signalled by certain demographic and historical features of the patient's case, most importantly, a history of previous violence.

Define specific aspects of the risk(s)

Having become concerned that there is a risk, the psychiatrist should:

- define the risk and estimate the *seriousness* of the potential harm
- make an estimate of the *probability* that the risk will become reality
- estimate the *imminence* that the risk will become reality.

Formulate a management plan to reduce risk(s)

Such a plan will utilize the detailed account of the risk behaviour in terms of the nature of the act, circumstances, the victim(s), precipitating factors, and substance misuse to inform risk-reducing interventions. Note the importance of an explicit time-scale.

Practical risk assessment

Assessments will vary according to the case and circumstances. Those undertaken to decide on a transfer from a maximum security hospital to one of medium security will differ from an assessment carried out in the emergency clinic on an unknown man who has been behaving oddly in public. It is not only a question of the differing resources and information available. The purposes of the assessments, the relative urgency of the decisions to be taken, and the period for which such decisions will hold sway are completely distinct.

The practical process of risk assessment can be thought of as having three stages: gathering and reviewing all documentation from all possible sources; examining the patient and interviewing informants; and asking yourself questions concerning the patient, the circumstances, and potential victims. From the documentation and interviews the psychiatrist aims to gain as complete a picture as possible of the index behaviour and its immediate antecedents; the patient's recent and longer term history, the patient's social and physical environment (with recent changes), and the patient's mental state. Close attention should to be paid to those areas where there are discrepancies between the patient's own account of his history and behaviour and those of other observers, particularly nursing staff.

The index behaviour

Frequently, risk assessment is required for patients who have already been violent or have threatened violence. In such cases it is of the utmost importance to record a detailed account of the index behaviour. The patient will provide a partial picture which may significantly minimize the violence. Any objective description is of great value, particularly witness statements recorded by the police. In addition to enabling analysis of the violent behaviour, witness statements often give a sharp and immediate sense of the emotional impact of the behaviour, an impact which is readily lost as the story is repeated through successive hospital admissions.

Such an account of the index behaviour may provide clues to the prevailing mental state which are otherwise unavailable. Psychosis may be suggested by disorganized behaviour, apparent responding to hallucinations, or bizarre actions. The patient may appear angry, afraid, or lacking in emotional response. His actions may appear planned, impulsive, or a response to frustration. He may have used a weapon defensively or with grossly excessive violence.

The immediate and medium-term antecedents

The immediate antecedents of the index violence may suggest precipitating factors. The patient may have suffered or be threatened by the loss of someone important. He may have experienced rejection. His accommodation or financial security may be at risk. He may have refused medication or increased his misuse of drugs or alcohol. Evidence of relapse may be evident without obvious cause. A pattern of change may be evident in the patient's life culminating in the index offence. He may have become increasingly socially isolated and withdrawn or have moved home ever more frequently, staying settled for increasingly short periods of time. Such 'social restlessness' has been seen as an ominous sign in the histories of particular psychotic perpetrators of irrational violence.

History

A comprehensive psychiatric history is an essential part of all risk assessments with additional attention paid to certain specific domains.

- *Previous violent behaviour* of each incident should be described. All behaviour bringing the patient into contact with the police should be ascertained, with the outcome recorded in terms of charge, conviction, and sentence including details of time spent in custody. Violent and criminal behaviour that did not come to police attention should also be recorded from as early as possible in the individual's life. So-called 'domestic violence' should not be neglected. Patterns, for example escalation in seriousness or decline in frequency should be noted.

- *Exposure to violence* of the patient, both as victim and witness, should be documented from the earliest stage of his developmental history and should include experiences 'in care'. While the mechanism is ill-understood, victims of abuse are at increased risk of becoming perpetrators in their turn.

- *Psychiatric career* of the patient should be reconstructed with attention to such factors as: mode of presentation; previous diagnostic formulations; whether admissions to hospital have been against the patient's will (under the Mental Health Act); the nature, efficacy, and time course of response to therapeutic intervention; and the various facets of insight including acceptance of medical explanations and advice, compliance with treatment, and spontaneously seeking psychiatric help. The success of outpatient management or the reasons for its failure are of particular importance. It may become clear that there is a constant relationship between psychiatric illness and violence and aggression or, on the other hand, that there is no relationship whatsoever.

- *Alcohol and drug misuse* history must be taken in detail, with particular attention to the relationships between drug use and psychiatric illness and between drug use and violence and aggression. These may be multiple and complex, for example violence when intoxicated may precede mental illness; drug use may exacerbate pre-existing psychotic symptoms associated with violence or precipitate relapse leading to violence; increased drug use may be an attempt by the patient to 'treat his symptoms'; criminal activity to finance a drug habit may follow loss of employment as a result of psychiatric illness.

- *Psychosexual and relationship* history should be explored in detail. Childhood experience of sexual abuse significantly increases the chances that the adult will become a perpetrator. A pattern of short unsuccessful intimate relationships may indicate one of a range of disorders of personality. Some understanding of attitudes to the opposite sex and sexual fantasies should be sought. Sexual psychopathology including dysfunction or abnormal sexual preference should be noted, especially if the latter has been acted upon outside a consensual relationship. Sexual partners are relatively frequent victims of severe violence associated with mental disorder, particularly if pathological jealousy is involved, and a pattern may be discernible over a series of relationships.

Circumstances

Thought should be given to how the patient's situation contributed to the index behaviour. Who was he in contact with? Was the behaviour of friends or family a factor, for example by encouraging drug or alcohol use or by discouraging compliance with treatment? Did the pattern of the patient's daily activities make the index behaviour more likely? Was the patient's accommodation appropriate?

The question of why the patient s victim was originally involved must be addressed. Was the victim a stranger, an acquaintance, or a family member? Was the victim selected as an individual, a member of a category, or at random?

Mental state

Just as a potentially suicidal patient should be asked about self-harm, so a potentially violent patient should be questioned explicitly about his intentions. He should be asked about specific victims (especially if threats have been made), methods, and plans.

Particularly associated with violence in psychosis are delusions of being under threat, of being controlled, and of having one's will over-ridden by some outside force. Acting on delusions is more likely if the delusions are associated with fear, suspicion, anger, or perplexity. Threats made by the patient must be taken seriously, as should violent fantasies. This applies as much to patients manifesting profound depression suggesting their families would be better off dead as to threats to kill uttered in anger.

The patient's insight should be examined in terms of his acceptance that he is ill, his agreement to take medication, and his understanding of the true nature of his psychotic experiences. Relative lack of conviction as to the truth of a delusion should not be seen as reassuring, since acting on false beliefs may be more likely if they are shakily rather than firmly held. Complete denial of the index violence or denial of personal responsibility for it are of ominous significance, as is a lack of remorse. The patient's attitude to any treatment he has received should be noted.

Relevant features of the patient's personality should be assessed. Personality strengths, such as the ability to make friends or cope stoically with adversity, may reduce risk. Deviousness or deceptiveness increase uncertainty. The damage to the personality frequently seen in schizophrenia may, in some cases, reduce the risk of violence by diminishing spontaneous activity. On the other hand, such patients actions are more difficult to predict because of reduced access to their mental state.

Risk assessment

Synthesis

Defining the seriousness of the potential harm, the probability it will occur, and its imminence, requires making sense of an often considerable amount of information. Patterns should be sought in the patient's development as a child, an adolescent, and an adult which will contribute to a complex picture of the patient, his circumstances, and his interaction with his potential victim. Prediction is facilitated by comparing and contrasting this picture with that of other patients with similar diagnoses, both known to the clinician personally and in the research literature.

Risk management

The purpose of risk assessment in psychiatry is the prevention of future harm by appropriate intervention. An effective strategy will change those aspects of the patient's situation and mental state which require changing and can be changed. It will also take into account important influences on behaviour, such as brain damage, which are not susceptible to intervention. Most importantly, the effects of each intervention should be monitored. Thus, long-term risk management involves a continuous process of risk assessment followed by intervention, followed by re-assessment of risk which either confirms risk reduction or indicates that the intervention has been unsuccessful. In other words, patient management is continuously subject to *feedback monitoring*.

Strategy and tactics for the management of patients who pose significant risk should be determined by the *multidisciplinary team*, especially by those individuals who will have specific roles in the patient's management. Success depends on the effective functioning of the team and on the *clear apportioning of responsibilities* within the team. Poor *communication* both within the team and between the team and other involved agencies has been held responsible for failures of management and the tragedies that have ensued.

Effective risk management involves breaking down a single large decision into a series of smaller steps. Thus, to decide that a given patient is unlikely to attack anyone before he is seen in the clinic a fortnight hence is a realistic possibility, whereas accurately predicting whether or not he will be safe in the indeterminate future is much less so. This patient's situation in the community, in terms of friends and family as well as support services, can only be reliably predicted in the short term.

Plans should be made to cover such eventualities as can be foreseen. These should be written down and made known to the relevant members of the team. As stated above, all plans should include provision for effective monitoring so that both successful and failed interventions can be noted. Appropriate responses in the event of the failure should be clearly spelt out. It is obvious that risk-management plans must take account of what is available locally, but it is equally obvious that plans may break down if a necessary minimum of community resources is unavailable.

8
Special problems

Childhood autism

This consists of a combination of impairments in social relationships, communication, and the development of imaginative interests. The most distinctive aberrations are the difficulties they show
in reciprocal social interaction, understanding the mental states of
other people, sharing their interests, and forming friendships and
intimate relationships. Their language lacks the usual social
quality, and is preoccupied with idiosyncratic concerns. It may be
lacking in quantity — for example, used only to ask for needs to
be met — or it may be plentiful but repetitive and more of a
monologue than a conversation. Pronoun reversal (for example,
'you' for 'me'), delayed echolalia, and stereotypical speech are
common features when language is reasonably well developed.
(Immediate echolalia is seen, but is also very common in simple
language delays and in children who are just learning to talk.) A
restricted and repetitive range of interests and behaviours is very
typical, and life may be dominated by incessant rituals, and distress and rage if trivial aspects of daily routine or environment are
changed. Partial forms of the disorder exist; the full form is
usually very persistent. Long-term advice and supervision are
needed, and families need support. Specialized educational
resources can be recommended; behaviour therapy techniques can
promote communicative development and reduce unacceptable
and challenging behaviours.

Hyperkinetic disorder

This is a combination of impairments, involving: an excess of
activity, especially in situations expecting calm; inattentive and
disorganized activity in every situation; and an 'impulsive' unwillingness to wait for gratification, share with others, or take one's

turn. A behavioural approach, with particular emphasis on speed of reinforcement, can be helpful both at home and in school. Drug treatment, especially with stimulants such as methylphenidate or dexamphetamine, is a powerful way of reducing hyperactive behaviour; and is therefore used in selected cases to promote social adjustment.

Specific developmental disorders

These occur when there is an impairment of one or more developmental functions markedly out of keeping with the general level of development. For some functions there are reliable and valid tests that have norms for different ages: specific reading retardation, for example, occurs when performance on a standard reading test is worse than the 5th centile, allowing for age and IQ; and it should be diagnosed by a psychologist's quantitative assessment. For other mental abilities, for example calculating, norms are much less satisfactory. For others again, such as motor delays and impairments of memory and attention, the diagnosis still has to be made on the basis of the clinical assessment. For all these problems, remedial education can be given once the problem is recognized. Counselling the child and the family will probably be needed to help in the prevention of secondary psychiatric dysfunction (see pp. 44–9).

Suicidal thoughts

Definitions

- *Suicide* is a wilful self-inflicted life-threatening act which has resulted in death.

- *Parasuicide* is a non-fatal act in which an individual deliberately causes self-injury or ingests a substance in excess of any prescribed or generally recognized therapeutic dose.

- *Deliberate self-harm* (DSH) is a deliberate non-fatal act committed in the knowledge that it was potentially harmful and, in the case of drug overdosage, that the amount taken was excessive.

Note that in definitions 2 and 3, the presence of *suicide intent* is not required. The term *attempted suicide* should no longer be used since it implies the presence of *suicidal intent.*

Assessment

Assess for:

- risk of suicide
- risk of repetition of DSH
- presence of psychiatric disorder
- current problems/events/coping resources including social support.

Features in the history associated with increased suicide risk

- any psychiatric history (especially schizophrenia, depression, and drug/alcohol dependence)
- recent discharge from hospital forensic history, previous DSH
- impulsive personality traits, social isolation (divorced > widows > never married)
- recent bereavement, painful physical illness
- older age (but rates rise amongst young men!)
- male sex
- unemployment
- low social class
- suicidal behaviour in environment
- easy access to means (anaesthetists, gun owners, drug users)
- certain professions (doctors, vets, farmers)
- certain 'minority' groups (Indian women; Irish people)
- epilepsy.

Also assess for the presence of *protective factors*:

- children or other dependents at home
- sometimes, religious convictions.

Mental state features associated with increased suicide risk

Assess for:

- presence of suicidal ideation
- hopelessness
- depression
- agitation
- early schizophrenia with retained insight (young patients who see their ambitions restricted)
- presence of delusions of control, poverty, guilt.

Assess DSH-act to estimate risk of repetition and suicide

Check for:

- Degree of planning/impulsivity
- performance in isolation or in front of others
- likeliness of being found in time
- precautions taken (e.g. no appointments made)
- attendance at hospital (A&E) of own volition
- quantity of tablets taken (all tablets available or only some)
- expectations of outcome irrespective of medical seriousness
- was a suicide note left? (if so, what did it say?)

Precipitating factors

Check for conflicts in areas of relationships, employment, finances, law/police, housing, sexual adjustment, physical health (especially HIV), bereavement.

Relevant resources

Assess the social support available, previous coping skills (help-seeking). Is there a good relationship with the general practitioner?

Alcohol and drinking problems

Although acknowledged to be an important part of the psychiatric examination, the drinking history is often overlooked or patchy. Clinicians may feel that they are inadequately trained and too busy, or may perceive individuals with alcohol problems as 'too difficult' and time consuming. This view can be reinforced by the frequent attendance of severely alcohol dependent individuals in crisis — intoxicated, aggressive, or suicidal. Taking an alcohol history is not the mere assimilation of facts; it is an opportunity to form a therapeutic relationship with the patient, may diffuse a difficult situation, and may even be helpful in itself.

Rather than confronting the patient with questions on quantity consumed and frequency of consumption at the outset, and risking a defensive reply, it may be more helpful to open with a non-specific question such as what they perceive as the main problem.

The alcohol history in the context of the background history

Ask about:

- *Family history*: family attitudes to alcohol; whether alcohol was kept in the house; the drinking history of parents, significant others and siblings; family history of alcohol and other psychiatric problems.
- *Personal history*: birth history; reached and when; school attendance and performance; peer relationships; truancy; educational attainment.
- *Occupational history*: what occupation — whether this involves working with alcohol; occupational problems related to alcohol (dismissal, absenteeism, frequent job changes).

- *Sexual and marital history*: sexual problems; history of childhood sexual abuse (particularly important in women with alcohol problems); HIV risk behaviour; marital problems related to drinking; separation; divorce; problems with children.

- *Financial and housing history*: housing problems; rent arrears; eviction; problems with neighbours.

- *Forensic history*: convictions for drink-driving; being drunk and disorderly; violent behaviour.

- *Past medical and psychiatric history*: particular attention should be paid to alcohol-related physical and psychological problems and accidents. Specific enquiry should be made for depressive illness, phobic anxiety, pathological jealousy, suicide attempts, and drug misuse.

- *Basic personality*: Ask the patient to describe what they were like before they developed their drinking problem.

Drinking history

Evolution of drinking and current alcohol consumption

Age of:

- first drink
- regular weekend drinking
- regular evening drinking
- regular lunchtime drinking
- early morning drinking.

Ascertain consumption at each stage, noting type of beverage and quantity consumed, as well as frequency. Note whether they prefer to drink in a group, alone in a social setting, or alone at home. Note whether there is any binge drinking and detail any periods of abstinence.

Obtain alcohol consumption (units) for the past 24 hours, 6 months, and 12 months (1 unit = 8–10 g of alcohol = 1 glass of wine/half-pint of ordinary strength beer/1 measure of spirits).

Evolution of alcohol dependence

Note age of onset of withdrawal symptoms and other features of the alcohol dependence syndrome (ICD-10):

- compulsion to drink
- difficulties in controlling alcohol consumption
- tolerance
- progressive neglect of alternative pleasures or interests
- persisting with drinking despite clear evidence of overtly harmful consequences.

Alcohol-related problems

Outline physical, neuropsychiatric, and social problems.

- *Physical*: gastritis, hepatitis, cirrhosis, pancreatitis, peptic ulcer, oesophageal varices, oesophageal carcinoma, seizures, cognitive impairment, peripheral neuropathy, cerebellar degeneration, anaemia, cardiomyopathy, myopathy, head injury, etc.
- *Neuropsychiatric*: memory blackouts, pathological intoxication, delirium tremens, depression, phobic anxiety, suicide attempts, pathological jealousy, personality change, sexual dysfunction, auditory hallucinations during withdrawal, alcoholic hallucinosis, eating disorders.
- *Social*: Marital/occupational and financial problems, forensic history.

A typical recent heavy-drinking day

Most patients can identify a typical recent heavy-drinking day. Some cannot, and this may imply more variability in their drinking, with a tendency perhaps to weekend binge drinking. Ask the patient to take you through the day from the moment of wakening. A description of the timing and consumption of the first drink, and the patient's attitude towards it can be extremely helpful in determining the degree of dependence. Thus, a man waking at 4.00 a.m., tremulous and drenched in sweat, who reaches out for the can of strong beer by the bed, is at a different stage of dependence from the man who takes his first drink at lunchtime. Likewise, the professional woman who drinks covertly from a bottle of vodka in a workplace lavatory at 9.00 a.m. is at a different stage from the woman who starts to drink at 5.00 p.m.

Other drug use

Has the patient ever used other drugs? (see next section.)

Treatment history

Was this provided by: GP; community alcohol team (statutory or voluntary); out-patient or in-patient treatment in general or psychiatric hospitals; residential rehabilitation; self-help group (AA)?

Drug dependence

When the answers to your screening questions, or other information (such as a routine urine drug screen), suggest that the patient has been using drugs, you will need to take a more detailed drug history. Below is a list of elements you will need to elicit, followed by a suggested schema, and some suggested questions.

Important elements of the history

- Which drug (s) is the patient using?
- What is the frequency of use?
- What is the pattern of a typical drug-using — day or week?
- What is the route of use (e.g. oral, smoked, snorted, injected)?
- What effect is the patient seeking when using the drug?
- Is there evidence of the physical or psychological features of dependence on the drug(s)?

- What risky behaviours does the patient engage in (e.g. injecting, sharing needles, unsafe sex, 'sex for drugs').

- How long is the history of drug use and how has it evolved?

- What complications of drug use has the patient experienced (physical, psychological, family, occupational and legal problems)?

- What is the patient's past experience of treatment for a drug problem? Have there been any periods of abstinence, and, if so, what has helped the patient to achieve this? What triggers have brought on relapses?

In addition, when you are taking a social history from the patient, assess the extent to which the patient's main social contacts are other drug users and whether there are friends, family, or others who do not use drugs and who could provide support.

Suggested schema for drug history

Current drug use

Which drugs does the patient currently use? Ask the patient to describe his or her drug use the previous day, and to take you through a typical drug-using day (which drug, how often, which route). Also ask about the circumstances of the drug use: for example, some people will only use drugs in certain social circumstances such as Ecstasy use at a dance party, while others may have a regular pattern of use which has developed to prevent the experience of withdrawal symptoms. Ask about a typical week if drugs are not used every day. Does the patient experience any withdrawal symptoms (ask the patient to describe them) or craving if the drug is not used? Ask about other symptoms of the dependence syndrome, such as increased tolerance to the drug, the priority of drug-seeking over other duties and pleasures withdrawal symptoms (ask the patient to describe them), or craving if the drug is not used. Is the patient currently engaging in any risky behaviour such as dangerous injecting (into groins or neck, or infected injection sites), sharing needles, or unsafe sex? How is he or she financing the drug use?

History of drug use

In addition to the current drug use, ask the patient if he or she has used other drugs in the past. If the patient has used more than one drug it is usually easier to take a chronological history of each drug in turn rather than to try to assess all of them at once.

Ask about the age at first use of the drug, then when the patient began to use the drug regularly. Ask about maximum frequency and amount used, and about any periods of abstinence. When (if ever) did the patient first experience withdrawal symptoms of the drug (ask the patient to describe them)? If not currently injecting, has the patient ever injected, and ever shared needles? Has the patient engaged in other risky behaviour (as above) in the past? What influences have helped the patient to achieve abstinence and then later to relapse?

Complications of drug use

Physical complications

Include complications of the drug itself and complications of the route of use. Ask specifically about hepatitis and HIV (for example: 'Have you ever worried that you might have caught hepatitis or HIV?', 'Have you had any tests?'). Also ask about other complications of injecting such as abscesses, deep vein thromboses, and septicaemia. Has the patient ever overdosed accidentally?

Psychological complications

Ask about the relationship of psychological symptoms to drug use. It may be difficult to tease out cause and effect, but some initial information will help in your assessment.

Family, occupational, and legal complications

Ask the patient about the effect of drug use upon these areas of his or her life.

Treatment history

Ask about previous experiences of seeking help for a drug problem. Has the patient had help from a GP, drug dependency unit or non-NHS organization? What has it involved: for instance, has the patient received prescriptions, or previous detoxification, or psychological treatment, or self-help? What does the patient think was helpful in the past?

Current wishes and intentions

There are several possible goals in the treatment of drug misusers. Abstinence is one possible goal, but safer drug use may be a more realistic target for some drug users (see Chapter 10, p. 198). Ask the patient what he or she would like to do about the drug use.

Special points in the physical examination

In the physical examination, look for injection sites, including legs and groins. If the patient is injecting, ask him or her to show you the most recent injection sites. Look for abscesses or infected sinuses, and for evidence of deep vein thrombosis for treatment, see p. 197.

Checklist of information

By the end of the history, you should have enough information to know:

- whether the patient is a dependent drug user
- what risks he or she is taking in relation to drug use, and
- whether there are current problems related to drug use.

Sexual and relationship problems

Sexual dysfunctions and desire disorders

History

This is taken from both partners separately, at least in part, but much of it can be usefully obtained from a joint interview, which also affords the possibility of direct observation of the couple.

Features include:

Nature and duration of the problem — is it a disorder of desire or of function?

- when was the last successful experience?
- does the problem occur in all situations (e.g. with other partners or in self-stimulation) or is it confined to the present relationship?
- does it occur at all attempts — if not, what proportion of the time?
- factors that seem to make it better or worse
- reaction of patient and partner when the problem occurs
- any associated difficulty (e.g. anorgasmia in the woman accompanying premature ejaculation)
- attempts to treat the problem so far (both in therapy and by couple's own initiative).

Associated factors — ask about e.g. alcohol intake, smoking, spinal injuries, diabetes, hypertension, psychiatric illness and its medication, physical illness, surgical operations, stress, prior traumatic experiences (including sexual abuse or rape), recent life events, life cycle stage, etc.; Quality of general relationship — ask about communication, resentment, inhibitions, distance and closeness, invalidism, power, commitment.

Any infidelities, satisfaction with sexual life, problems with fertility; duration of present relationship, sexual preferences and practices, inhibitions? History from each partner — include questions regarding sexual development, previous relationships and sexual experience, attitudes of family to sex, levels of knowledge, puberty, menarche, obstetric history, contraception, menopause, HRT, pelvic injuries or surgery, any sexual deviations, effects of ageing:

Full biographical and family history — often obtained via a self-report questionnaire before the couple are seen. This should include family history, personal history, relationships and children, personality assessment and a general symptom checklist.

Masturbation (past and present) — attitudes, guilt, fantasies, techniques, etc. Is orgasm achieved? Physical examination is desirable although not essential in all cases, but it is usually recommended in cases of erectile disorder and vaginismus.

Diagnostic features

The problems presenting in the male partner are: erectile disorder (impotence); premature ejaculation; delayed ejaculation; loss of desire.

Those presenting in the female partner are: vaginismus; orgasmic dysfunction; dyspareunia (pain during intercourse); and loss of desire.

Problems deriving from the relationship include incompatibility of sexual desire and conflict over sexual preferences and practice.

Direct questions should be asked about the presence of morning or night erections (suggesting a psychogenic aetiology), alcohol intake, use of drugs, sources of stress, any psychiatric problems, diabetes, hypertension, spinal injuries, pelvic injuries or operations, genitourinary infections, etc.

There are no diagnostic tests which need to be performed in cases of ejaculatory or orgasmic dysfunctions, but medication with SSRIs or other antidepressant drugs should be queried.

In erectile dysfunction there are some basic points which should be addressed. Enquiry should be made into the use of medication, including antidepressants, diuretics, gastric acid suppressants, and antihypertensives. Arterial blood pressure is a useful measure, as are reflexes in the lower limb and cremasteric reflexes, penile sensitivity, blood or urine sugar levels, and examination of the genitals. In erectile disorders the best source of information (if the test is available) is the intracavernosal injection of papaverine or prostaglandin: if an erection can be produced by this means it excludes vascular causes, but leaves open the differentiation between psychogenic and neurogenic causation. This has to be determined on clinical grounds, but it is often necessary to assume a multifactorial causation. Further tests, including arteriograms and cavernosograms, should be reserved for those cases in which surgery is being contemplated.

In problems of sexual desire in men there is some benefit to be obtained from the measurement of hormone levels, especially of testerosterone, dihydrotestosterone, luteinizing hormone, follicle stimulating hormone, sex hormone binding globulin and prolactin.

In cases of vaginismus a digital examination of the vagina is necessary to make the diagnosis, but in many centres this is done at a later visit, when the patient is more comfortable with the setting.

Sexual deviations and gender dysphoria

History

Denial is a common phenomenon in those with sexual deviations. In order to obtain a truthful account it is useful to ask open questions and to approach the topic in a roundabout way. For example, a man with tendencies to abuse children will probably not disclose this immediately, but if asked about hobbies or interests he will give clues to his preferences and may eventually be quite frank and open about them.

Elicit from the patient:

Details of the deviant behaviour: how often does this occur, where, when, with whom, whether caught and/or convicted, whether fantasies are associated, etc.

What thoughts and feelings are experienced? What visual images or materials are used to achieve arousal? Does the person have a normal sexual outlet as well as the deviant one? What are the masturbatory fantasies?

How high is the sexual drive (may be judged by masturbatory frequency or desired frequency of ejaculation)?

How dangerous is the activity? Is it against the law? Does it damage the patient or others? Is there any empathy with possible victims?

Do family members or partner know about the activities? What is their attitude?

Is there a past criminal history (this problem or others)?

Is the patient motivated by the wish to change his behaviour or simply to avoid punishment?

Is there an associated sexual dysfunction in more 'normal' sexual activities?

In cases of *gender dysphoria* has there been a wish to be a member of the opposite sex from childhood, or is it more recent in origin? Has it occurred in the course of a depressive or psychotic illness? Has the patient thought through all the implications of sex change for themselves, their family, and friends?

Diagnostic features

Variations and deviations can be divided into those which are harmful to others and those which are either solitary or harmless. Deviant sexual behaviour is predominantly a male problem, but it should be remembered that, especially with child abuse, women can also be perpetrators.

Harmful deviations include: sexual abuse of children, whether general (paedophilia) or confined to family members (incest); rape (heterosexual or homosexual); indecent assault; exhibitionism; voyeurism; obscene telephone calls; stalking; frotteurism (touching people sexually in crowds); stealing clothing (to use fetishistically); and the more dangerous forms of sadomasochism including sex–murder.

Solitary deviations include: cross-dressing for the purpose of sexual arousal; auto-erotic asphyxia; and various forms of fetishism, including leather, rubber, shoes, underclothes, or different parts of the body such as feet. Relatively harmless deviations include cross-dressing for sexual arousal in the presence of the partner, the use of fetishistic objects with the partner, and some of the more benign forms of sadomasochism such as domination–submission, bondage, and spanking.

Transsexualism is not usually defined as a deviation, but is included here because there seems no more suitable place to discuss it. There are generally no biological abnormalities in these patients, for treatment, see p. 207.

Couple relationship therapy

History

This is not usually a major part of couple therapy, and in some centres it is elicited by prior completion of a questionnaire by each partner. What is required is a basic version of the general psychiatric history, including: presenting problems; and (for both partners) family history; personal history; previous relationships; current relationship; children; personality; and a brief symptom checklist.

In more psychodynamic settings the history comes out gradually in the course of therapy. Some systemic therapists spend time with 'genograms' or diagrammatic family trees to help understand family influences, see p. 47. In most clinics the therapist is as interested in the observed interaction of the couple in therapy as in the history itself.

In the couple interview, therapists will elicit details of the presenting problem, other strains in the relationship, the general satisfaction and commitment of both partners, the good aspects and troublesome aspects of the relationship, the risk of divorce or separation, problems with children, housing and financial problems, sexual satisfaction, and what attracted them to each other.

Have there been major quarrels or violence? Infidelity? What are the resentments on both sides? Do they confide in each other? Who is more upset by the current problems?

Diagnostic features

These are more concerned with the couple relationship than the individual, and involve such factors as closeness–distance, dominance–submission, alliances and boundaries, repetitive sequences of interaction, role-taking by each partner, relationships with other family members and outsiders.

Observation of the interaction will reveal other aspects of the relationship. Who is the natural spokesperson? Who defers to the other's opinion? Who is labelled as the sick or abnormal one? Who interrupts the other one? How are conflicts initiated, escalated, and solved? Do they communicate clearly or obscurely? Do they understand each other or are there clear miscommunications? Does one make jokes at the other's expense? Which partner is more committed and/or more possessive? Do the partners respect each other's views and opinions? Can they show empathy? Do they share a sense of humour? Do they continue to raise issues from the past? Can they negotiate differences? What are the attraction factors in the relationship? What are the strengths?

Eating disorders

History

Many sufferers of eating disorders feel extremely ashamed about what they are doing and may find your questions very taxing and painful. Others are ambivalent about whether they want help, in some cases the denial is so extreme that they feel there is little or nothing wrong with them, and they have merely come to the clinic because of extreme concerns by their family or partner. Especially in these latter cases it is important to establish an individual relationship with the patient rather than to relate exclusively to the family.

These patients arouse strong feelings, which range from anger and irritation through to the desire to rescue and protect. This is probably because their interpersonal schema include a mixture of a drive to please others, a sense of inferiority, and a drive to be in control. One of the most important parts of the management of these patients is to understand this transference and counter-transference.

Behavioural assessment

At the simplest behavioural level, by the end of the assessment interview the clinician wants to know the following:

- Is severe undernutrition present or is the patient significantly overweight?

- Is there constant dietary restriction and/or are there episodes of overeating?

- What weight control measures are used?

These behavioural criteria are easy to define and elicit, but they are also of clinical utility since they guide management.

Under-nutrition or overweight?

This is addressed by measuring weight and height and is usually performed at the end of the interview as part of the physical examination (see below). A detailed lifetime weight and diet history is helpful. The patient should be asked when she first noticed a problem with her weight or when she first began to focus on weight as a topic of personal importance. Both the **rate** of weight loss and the **absolute level** are markers of dangerousness. Marked fluctuations suggest that there is self-induced vomiting or abuse of laxatives and diuretics.

The patient should be asked what her heaviest ever weight was, and when this occurred, and similarly about her lowest weight. Her weight when her periods began needs to be established as does the weight at which her periods stopped (if relevant). This is important as the weight at which the patient's normal biological functions recover will generally be slightly above the former and so can give an indication of how much weight needs to be gained.

It is also useful to obtain a family weight history. There may be a strong family history of obesity in bulimia nervosa or of leanness or eating disorder in anorexia nervosa.

Constant dietary restriction and/or episodes of overeating?

It is often necessary to question about bulimic behaviour directly as it may not be mentioned spontaneously because of the shame attached. A suitable line of enquiry is: 'Do you have episodes when your eating seems excessive or out of control'. You need to probe gently to elicit whether the amount eaten is excessive (objective binge > 1000 kcalories) or not (subjective binge).

What weight control measures are used?

In addition to dietary restriction the commonly employed methods are: self-induced vomiting; chewing and spitting; abuse of laxatives; diuretics; street drugs (for example, amphetamines and ecstasy); caffeine; prescribed medication such as thyroxine; or health-food preparations; excessive exercise.

Mental state assessment

Overvalued ideas about shape and weight, in which the assessment of self-worth is made exclusively in these terms, are considered primary features of bulimia nervosa. Not all patients with anorexia nervosa express such ideas.

Body image distortion (a statement that they are fat when, in fact, they are underweight) is no longer regarded as a necessary criteria for anorexia nervosa. A less culturally bound description of this phenomenon is that the emaciated state is overvalued.

The patient should also be asked what weight she would ideally like to be. Often patients with anorexia nervosa will try to please the therapist by giving a higher weight than they are aiming for. It maybe helpful to probe into this in some detail: 'If you got to seven stone (44.5 kg) would you be happy there?' If the patient says 'No' it can be helpful to press her, as this may help her realize that she has a problem: 'So if you were seven stone you might want to weigh six and a half, but what then?'

Additional psychiatric disorders

Over 80 per cent of people with eating disorders have additional psychiatric morbidity during the course of their life. Depression and obsessional symptoms are common in anorexia nervosa. Depression and anxiety disorders are common in bulimia. Symptoms of post-traumatic stress disorder are common in mixed anorexia nervosa and bulimia nervosa.

Personality disorders are present in 50 per cent of cases referred to specialist centres.

Diagnostic features to look out for:

- body mass index less than 17.5 kg/m^2
- use of weight control measures
- spot diagnosis–physical signs, such as parotid or submandibular gland enlargement, eroded teeth, 'Russell's sign' callus on back of hand, cold blue hands; lanugo hair.

Body mass index can be calculated as follows:

$$\frac{\text{Weight (in kilograms)}}{\text{height} \times \text{height (in metres)}}$$

Physical assessment

Nutrition

For many patients it is very difficult to allow themselves to be weighed. It is important not to get drawn into a battle over this and the greater the weight of the patient the more lenient you can afford to be. The ICD-10 definition of anorexia nervosa requires that the body mass index is less that 17.5 kg/m^2 (this approximates well to the DSMIV definition of 15 per cent below average weight).

Cardiovascular system

The hands, feet, and nose are pinched, blue, and cold. In severe cases chilblains and, particularly in children, gangrene of the toes can occur. The pulse rate is slow (less than 60) and blood pressure is low at 90/60. A marked fall in blood pressure on standing (postural drop) is evidence of dehydration.

Skin and hair

The skin is dry and downy, lanugo hair may be present on the cheeks, nape of the neck, and forearms and legs. The head hair may become thinned and dry so that it breaks off and sticks out. There may be a scar over the knuckles (Russell's sign) if the hand is used to induce vomiting. A petechial rash due to thrombocytopenia can occur with severe starvation.

Gastrointestinal system

Vomiting can lead to many physical consequences. The teeth may appear small and smooth with the upper front teeth worn into an arch shape; alternatively, the teeth may be deceptively even if they have been crowned. The side of the mouth may be cracked. The face may appear rounded due to swelling of the salivary glands.

Skeletomuscular system

A proximal myopathy develops in severe cases. If this is present the patient may find lifting her arms to brush her hair difficult. She may not be able to get up without help or without leverage from her arms if you ask her to crouch. Tetany can develop because of the metabolic alkalosis (common in vomiting), for treatment, see p. 214.

Somatization

Definition

Somatization is the term given when patients who fulfil criteria for a psychological disorder (usually depression and/or anxiety) believe instead that they have a physical condition. This is a very common presentation of psychiatric disorder and is neither abnormal nor unusual. Somatization disorder refers to the most severe cases, and is a diagnostic category to describe patients who report large numbers of somatic symptoms, have illness histories stretching back to adolescence, and are very frequent users of medical services. The disorder is uncommon, but very demanding in terms of cost and time.

Taking a history from a patient with severe somatization can be difficult if one is a psychiatrist. The intention is to obtain the usual information on the mental state, but without challenging the patient or becoming too 'psychological'. Thus do not ask: 'Are you depressed?', but 'Has all this got you down'. Do not ask: 'Do you feel like killing yourself', but: 'Have all your problems ever got too much for you', and so on. Do not ask: 'Do you get panic attacks', but instead probe about whether or not certain situations, such as supermarkets or the underground, make the patient worse.

The patient who tells you they are made worse by neon lights, or whose 'brain gets overloaded by lots of conversations going on at once' may be experiencing phobic-related symptoms. Stress is a term that is often acceptable to patients when more direct psychological approaches fail.

One of the most important questions is: 'What do you think is wrong with you?'. The patient's illness model may explain much of their behaviour, as well as pointing to possible treatment avenues. Someone who is worried that when they get back pain their 'disc will slip again' and they will end up in a wheelchair will naturally restrict their activities. Many have similar 'catastrophic' cognitions — 'If I push myself I may never walk again, or I'll have a relapse'. Always ask: 'What might happen if you continued (when you get the pain … feel exhausted … feel dizzy)' and: 'What is the worst thing that might happen to you?'.

The history

The medical and family history of patients with chronic somatization can be revealing. A history of previous unexplained symptoms is common — tonsillitis persisting after the complete removal of tonsils — 'grumbling appendix' — prolonged recovery from normal infections — repeated gynaecological procedures, and so on. Illness may also run in the family — looking after parents with long-term illnesses (either physical or psychological) is common. Previous episodes of ill-defined illnesses, such as candida or unusual allergies, are suggestive.

Always take a history of previous contacts with the medical profession — it is not advisable to criticize medical colleagues, but allow the patient to ventilate their distress at what may have been very unsatisfactory previous encounters.

Course

Somatization disorder is, by definition, a chronic condition. Patients attending specialist clinics with labels such as ME or chronic fatigue syndrome also have a gloomy outlook, associated with the strength of their physical illness convictions and the degree of avoidance behaviour.

Investigations

In general, most patients will already have had more than enough investigations. Once basic sensible investigations have been performed, further investigations will reinforce the sense that something organic is wrong. Investigations do not reassure such patients, and are anxiogenic, not anxiolytic. A better use of your time is to obtain as many medical records as you can, (for treatment, see p. 205).

Mother and baby problems

Pregnancy

Most general psychiatrists, at some time or another, will look after pregnant patients, and a detailed assessment of the mother's mental health and adjustment may be necessary for a variety of purposes or reasons (discussed below). Maternal psychopathology in pregnancy is the same as psychopathology in other settings, thus the principles of detailed history-taking and systematic mental state evaluation are the same irrespective of childbearing status. The interviewer should, however, be sensitive to the fact that, in general, only a fortunate few expectant mothers conform to the stereotype of the pregnant woman who 'blooms' with good health; for many mothers early pregnancy is a time of tiredness, appetite changes, nausea, loss of libido, etc. There may be anxieties and concerns about the future, doubts about their readiness for parenthood, and uncertainties about the stability of key relationships, for example with the partner. Fears, ruminations, and fantasies about the foetus may have a bearing on the mother's mental state, but it may not be mentioned unless asked about and then only if the mother has confidence in the interviewer.

What is the personal and social context of the pregnancy — is it a first baby, have there been previous miscarriages and terminations? If it is a second or subsequent pregnancy how old are the other children, are they in good health, and is the mother anticipating problems with the arrival of the new child? How much help and support does she have from family and friends and how supportive is the expectant father financially, practically, and emotionally? What is his mental health like? Thus the context of pregnancy imparts a particular focus to the psychiatric examination, and, in terms of the mother's history, it becomes especially important to know what her own experience of being parented was like and what experience she has had of looking after babies and little children.

Clinically significant depression and anxiety is not uncommon in early pregnancy and may be missed unless specifically asked about. Clinical judgement is needed to distinguish between psychosomatic concomitants of depression and changes which occur in pregnancy. For example, can a woman who wakes up at night to micturate get back to sleep easily, does she wake feeling refreshed, is there a diurnal variation to her tiredness, and is her loss of appetite specific to certain kinds of foods? How does *she* construe her physical symptoms; that is to say, does she ascribe them to her pregnant condition?

Some important reasons for psychiatric examination in pregnancy

Termination of pregnancy

Abortion legislation varies greatly across nations and it is impossible to generalize about psychiatric indications. Suicidal risk and the possibility of severe post-partum destabilization of mental health are among the most prominent psychiatric considerations in countries with relatively restrictive abortion laws. There are no **absolute** psychiatric indications or contraindications to abortion (that is apart from religious, moral, and legal considerations), there are no psychiatric illnesses or indeed associated disorders (for example, severe mental impairment) in which a woman's right to choose may be over-ruled on medical/psychiatric grounds.

Management of severe mental illness during pregnancy

Questions often arise about the teratogenic effects of prescribed and non-prescribed drugs. What balance is there between the putative benefits of discontinuing medication and a flare-up of maternal illness? Clearly such questions can only be addressed in the light of a detailed knowledge of the mother's history and current state.

Concerns about the welfare of the fetus and future safety of parenting of the newborn

Risks to the foetus may arise through infection, nutritional deficit, drug exposure, deliberate self-harm, and lack of compliance with antenatal care programmes. Thus the assessment of the mother's condition, for example chronic schizophrenia, eating disorder, drug dependence, personality disorder, depression, or mental impairment, takes on an added urgency because of the risk to the unborn child, and this risk may enter the equation when assessing the need for compulsory treatment under the provisions of the Mental Health Act. Longer-term concerns about the motivation and safety of parenting of the newborn should begin to be addressed during pregnancy in conjunction with Social Services. The psychiatrist may be asked to carry out an evaluation of the mother's mental illness, its history and prognosis, and her ability to manage her life in her personal and social context. There may be an inherent conflict between the mother's rights and wishes to be the primary carer of her baby and the paramount need to ensure the child's welfare and safety.

Prevention and management of post-partum recurrence of mental illness

The likelihood of recurrence of severe mental illness (manic depressive and schizo-affective disorder, and possibly also paranoid psychosis) is high. Relapse rates of up to 50 per cent are described and, therefore, it is negligent not to plan ahead by liaising with obstetric and primary health-care services to plan possible admission. Recurrence rates of non-psychotic depressive disorders are about 20 per cent. Accurate and expert antenatal assessment by a psychiatrist is essential for planned management at a time when the mother is in repeated contact with clinical (obstetric and primary health-care) services. Motivation to change may be a major factor in helping some expectant mothers to alter patterns of behaviour; for example, drug use and abuse.

After childbirth

The same general principles that applied to psychiatric examination in pregnancy also apply after the birth of the child. Thus some kinds of pre-existing mental illness have high rates of recurrence but, in addition, childbirth itself is a major factor in provoking first onsets of both psychotic and non-psychotic affective disorder. There are three conditions, the names of which suggest a specific association with childbirth — maternity blues, postnatal depression, and post-partum or puerperal psychosis.

Maternity blues

These are near universal, short-lived episodes of emotional lability, typically occurring around the 4th and 5th day post-partum. The commonest picture is of dysphoria, but this may in some instances be mingled with or dominated by elation, prolixity, and overactivity. The blues themselves do not constitute an illness or syndrome; the two main points of clinical interest are the identification of the characteristics of those women who go on to develop postnatal depression, and the distinction between the 'benign' self-limiting mood changes of the blues from the sinister prodromal symptoms of impending affective psychosis.

Postnatal depression

The symptoms of postnatal depression are the same as those of depression in other settings, but, in addition, the women frequently report ruminations of inadequacy and guilt about their ability to be good or competent mothers. Sometimes they describe feelings of aggression and impulses to harm the infant which are very rarely acted upon, but which induce further self-blame. Thus the assessment of depression after childbirth should always incorporate sensitive questions about the mother's feelings concerning her baby and should extend to include obsessional ruminations and rituals as well as psychological and behavioural manifestations of anxiety; for example, irrational fears, social and agoraphobic behaviours.

Post-partum or puerperal psychosis

These are affective (manic, mixed, or psychotic depressive) disorders, sometimes with paranoid, hallucinatory symptoms as well, which have an acute onset, usually at the end of the first or during the second week after delivery. They are commonly described as coming on after a 'lucid' period of a few days; the affective illness is often very fluctuating and rapidly changing in its presentation, with swings of mood and sometimes co-existing manic and depressive symptoms. In addition, it is suggested that the presence of 'non-organic' confusion, namely perplexity and patchy disorientation, may be pathognomonic. It is entirely possible, however, that any subject who is in the early stages of acute psychotic breakdown may present in a similar way.

At the moment there are no treatments rationally based on aetiological hypotheses, thus the choice of drugs is based on a judgement of the predominant clinical picture. Repeated assessments may be necessary and too frequent changes of medication leading to poly-pharmacy should be avoided. Such assessments should also take into account possible risks to the infant if mother and baby are admitted together. Risks may arise through an impulse in response to hallucinations or delusions; for example, the baby is evil and possessed or it is immortal and is an angel. Another major source of risk is through disorganization and neglect because the mother's interactions are too disturbed; for example, she is manic or agitated. Her interactions may be diminished because she is retarded, or they may be inappropriate because she is chronically and severely impaired and lacking insight as part of a schizophrenic illness. In such circumstances, the psychiatric examination must synthesize the doctor's own evaluation of the mother's mental state and behaviour both alone and in the presence of the baby, with the observations of nurses and other members of the clinical team. Decisions about whether temporarily to nurse the mother and baby separately may have to be backed by compulsion under the provisions of the Mental Health Act. Similarly, decisions about when it is safe to reunite them must depend upon the psychiatrist's assessment of the mother's mental state, her insight, and compliance with necessary restrictions.

Some neuropsychiatric syndromes

Early-onset dementias

Creutzfeld–Jacob disease (CJD)

This is a rare, progressive dementia transmitted by infection with a prion (slow virus particle). Spongiform encephalopathy develops, possibly after a prodrome of anxiety or depression. Intellectual decline is followed by spasticity, ataxia, and myoclonic jerks. The terminal stage is of muteness and rigidity, with death occurring within two years. EEG may show a characteristic triphasic pattern. Treatment is palliative.

Pick's disease

Rare, probably hereditary dementia classically affecting the frontal lobes initially, but pathology also shows a knife-blade atrophy in the temporal lobes. Women > men. Presentation usually occurs between 50 and 60 years of age. Early symptoms are of personality change and selective speech disorder, and later other 'frontal' features as well as memory impairment become apparent. Neuroimaging (by MRI) reveals frontal and, sometimes, anterior temporal atrophy. Treatment includes genetic counselling

Huntington's disease

An autosomal dominant disorder (triple repeat on the short arm of Chromosome 4). Presentation is usually in the fourth decade of life, men = women. Insidious onset of involuntary choreiform movements affecting the face, head, and arms. Initially these can be disguised by the patient. Depression or explosive outbursts may occur. Later a progressive dementia and athetoid movements are evident. Disease duration is 12–16 years. Results of investigation include a 'flat' EEG and caudate atrophy on MRI. Early disease may be detected by looking for decreased metabolism in the caudate with functional neuroimaging. Treatment is low-dose haloperidol, or tetrabenazine.

Normal-pressure (communicating) hydrocephalus

Onset often occurs in later life, but this dementia is potentially reversible. Gait ataxia, cognitive impairment, urinary incontinence, and nystagmus are the clinical features. CSF pressure is normal most of the time, but imaging can reveal enlarged ventricles and cortical atrophy. Treatment is a ventriculoperitoneal shunt.

Parkinson's disease

The mean age of onset in this familial disorder is 55. Cogwheel rigidity, festinant gait, and bradykinesia are well known, but psychiatric features such as depression are very common. Also, anti-parkinsonian drugs are linked to a variety of psychiatric side-effects, especially psychotic and hallucinatory disorders. In the older patient, arteriosclerotic parkinsonism is frequent; cognitive impairment here is recognized and associated with the concentration of Lewy bodies. Management should involve liaison with a neurologist.

Amnesic (Korsakoff's) syndrome

Thiamine deficiency, CNS poisoning, or hippocampal damage are all causative. A retrograde amnesia (failure to recall events before the onset of the disorder) and anterograde amnesia (poor memory for events after the onset of the disorder) are present. There is impaired ability to learn and disorientation for time, but immediate recall is often preserved. Confabulation occurs, perhaps as the patient realizes there is a memory void, but is not diagnostic. There is no overall global cognitive decline. Treatment is for the underlying cause, but total recovery is exceptional.

CNS infections

Human immunodeficiency virus (HIV)

HIV dementia is now thought to be the commonest dementia in young people. It is of insidious onset with subtle impairment of memory and concentration being observed initially. Apathy and withdrawal, or social disinhibition also occur. Poor balance, dysarthria, and tremor can be found, but severe global decline and profound psychomotor retardation rapidly develop. Death due to opportunistic infection, aspiration pneumonia, etc., is the outcome within two years for 90 per cent of cases. Space-occupying lesions, such as lymphoma, are well recognized in HIV disease, and require treatment at a specialist unit. Delirium and a paranoid psychosis, as a result of HIV, are also reported. These are treated in the usual way. Adjustment disorders, anxiety, compulsive rituals, and depression are all found amongst the psychiatric sequelae of HIV diagnosis.

Neurosyphilis

Caused by *Treponema pallidum,* this is now a rare form of organic psychosis and dementia. Frontal lobe involvement is common, leading to personality change, and there is a gradual deterioration in memory and intellect. Depression is often a presenting feature. *Argyll–Robertson pupils* (small, irregular, and unreactive to light but not to accommodation) are seen in over 50 per cent of cases. Later, there is a lower limb weakness, resulting in a spastic paralysis. Serum and CSF Venereal Disease Research Laboratory (VDRL) and *T. pallidum* haemagglutination (TPHA) tests are positive. High-dose penicillin with steroid cover (to avoid the Herxheimer reaction) is the standard treatment.

Cerebrovascular disease

Cerebrovascular accident (or stroke)

Apart from the physical deficits resulting from stroke, depression is an important sequelae which can be overlooked; it is said to be more common in dominant anterior lesions. Treatment of choice is probably an SSRI antidepressant. Also, continuing hypertension or thromboembolic disease needs careful treatment as otherwise progressive cognitive impairment can result.

Subdural haematoma

Peak incidence occurs between 50 and 60 years of age. Effects are manifest weeks or months after the initial head injury (which may be trivial). First, persistent headache and, later, recurrent fluctuations in the level of consciousness are seen. Declining memory is usually obvious in longstanding cases and can be accompanied by neurological signs, such as ipsilateral weakness and hyperreflexia. Radioactive brain scan is diagnostic in 90 per cent of cases, and CT imaging is helpful. Surgical drainage is often indicated.

Subarachnoid haemorrhage

This is seen in 8 per cent of strokes, and results in high psychiatric morbidity. In addition to the early confusional state, personality change and anxiety are common. A difficulty with attention and concentration is seen rather than a decline in intelligence.

Head injury

Behavioural and psychosocial problems post-head injury are numerous and influential. The degree of post-traumatic amnesia and the Glasgow coma scale predict the severity of the head injury. A severe head injury leads to emotional and behavioural problems in about 70 per cent of cases, and these tend to manifest in the year after injury. Impaired self-control and impulsivity, as well as increased dependency and apathy are evident. There is difficulty learning from experience, even when new information is retained. Post-traumatic neurotic disorders, particularly anxiety and dysphoria, are seen. Special centres (such as Headway) exist for the severe cases.

Multiple sclerosis

Usually develops after childhood but before 50 years of age. Women are twice as likely to be affected as men, and there is sometimes a positive family history. Psychiatric features include persistent fatigue and depression. Cognitive decline occurs late in the disease, perhaps with associated euphoria. MRI shows white matter lesions or plaques, and visual-evoked potentials and CSF oligoclonal IgG are diagnostic.

9
When to refer to experts

Drug problems

You should feel able to ask for specialist advice whenever you do not feel confident with your management of a drug-using patient. However, specialist referral is suggested in the following particular circumstances:

- The patient requests specialist referral.
- The patient has features of the dependence syndrome.
- The patient has a complicated pattern of poly-drug use.
- The patient is pregnant.
- There is risky drug-using behaviour such as injecting.

Don't forget, however, to involve the general practitioner. Many GPs undertake basic substitute prescribing and are able to provide comprehensive care for their drug-using patients.

Alcohol problems

The following are indicators for specialist referral:

- severe dependence
- history of fits
- history of delirium tremens
- severe concurrent physical or mental illness (including cognitive impairment)
- repeated unsuccessful attempts at out-patient detoxification.

The following are medical emergencies requiring immediate hospital admission:

- delirium tremens
- Wernicke's encephalopathy.

Sexual and relationship problems

Sexual dysfunction and desire disorders

Referral of the couple is usually preferable, but individuals are accepted. Referrals of patients of any age from 16 upwards can be accepted. Heterosexual and homosexual individuals and couples can be treated. If a couple is referred, it is preferable for the relationship to be of at least a few months' duration.

Problems of desire, arousal (erection or penetration), and orgasm/ejaculation are appropriate for referral. It is better to deal with side-effects of drugs (for example, antidepressants or phenothiazines) before deciding to refer, as this can sometimes obviate the need for referral. Patient (and partner if there is one) should be well motivated for sex therapy.

The presence of organic factors such as diabetes or multiple sclerosis is not a contraindication to referral. In addition, the presence of depression, anxiety, or psychosis is not a contraindication to referral.

Sexual deviations and variations

These vary greatly in severity and in relevance, from very minor activities in an ongoing relationship to dangerous and harmful practices. Sexual variations within a relationship, for example mild sadomasochism and accepted transvestism, are probably not indications for referral.

Moderately severe deviations, such as exhibitionism, voyeurism, and frotteurism, could well merit referral to a behavioural–cognitive programme, to a forensic psychiatric clinic, or to a specialist forensic psychotherapy unit. In these cases it is important to establish the motivation of the patient for treatment, since those who are unmotivated for change, and those whose sole reason for accepting therapy is to avoid the involvement of the law, have a very poor prognosis in therapy.

More severe and damaging deviations, such as rape and child sexual abuse, are best dealt with by the forensic psychiatric services following a conviction: those who have not yet been apprehended but confess their activities to a psychiatrist present a problem as to when to break confidentiality. Advice should be sought from colleagues and/or Social Services and appropriate action taken to reveal the information in order to protect the public and prevent further crimes being committed.

Transsexualism and gender dysphoria

Although these can be treated in specialist clinics, there are very few in the UK. They require careful screening and should be referred only if there seems to be no doubt about the patient's motivation for gender reassignment and his/her ability to withstand the psychological and social pressures which may result.

Couple relationship problems

These are common both as relationship problems in themselves and in the context of many psychiatric difficulties, such as jealousy, depression, anxiety, and neuroses. Referral of all these and related problems is accepted by most couple therapy clinics. Referral of a couple or family is generally accepted, but referral of individuals is less acceptable in these clinics.

The more ill the patient, the more his family is also entitled to consideration, especially as they may be involved in the long-term care and support of the ill member. A great deal can be gained by making a family dynamic assessment the first step in establishing a suitable plan for assessment, investigation, and treatment of the index patient. Unfortunately, this is not always practical, for example in emergencies or when suitably skilled persons are not members of the treatment team. At present, referral to a family therapist is frequently a referral of last resort. In principle, any family who expresses a willingness to work together with a skilled professional in helping their ill member is suitable for referral for family therapy. In family therapy, no clear distinction is made between assessment and treatment: the first session aims to establish a treatment contract and this contract is reviewed regularly.

Many couple therapy clinics will also be able to carry out family therapy with older children in addition to the couple therapy: referral should state which family members are to be seen.

Couple problems are quite common where there has been a history of childhood trauma in one partner: these can be dealt with by a combination of couple and individual therapy.

Referral should be fully discussed with both partners and any other family members to be seen; agreement must be obtained from both or all prior to the referral. Most patients who are in a relationship can benefit from informally discussing the problem with their partner or other family members, with the help of the referring team, and it is worth while doing this before making a definitive referral to couple therapy.

Eating problems

Effective help is best provided by staff who understand eating disorders. Therefore, referral when the diagnosis is made is preferable. People with eating disorders find that being treated by someone who does not understand the condition is ineffective and may make the condition worse.

Consider emergency admission to a specialized unit for eating disorders or medical ward if:

- the body mass index (see p. 161) is less than 13.5 kg/m^2, especially if more than 25 per cent of body-weight lost in less than 6 months
- there is proximal myopathy
- there are signs of circulatory failure (pulse < 45; BP < 70/60 pre-gangrenous peripheries, frequent faints)
- there are signs of marrow failure, e.g. petechial haemorrhage
- there is a severe electrolyte imbalance (e.g. K < 2.5 mmol)
- there is hypoglycaemia.

Forensic psychiatry

Forensic psychiatry overlaps with all other psychiatric specialties. It is not a discrete area of psychiatry easily defined in terms of diseases, techniques, or age bands. All general psychiatrists, for example, will have in any current caseload a significant proportion of individuals with criminal records, and antisocial behavioural problems. From time-to-time, medico-legal reports will be requested on general psychiatric cases. These reports may be in relation to criminal charges, civil matters, such as compensation, or child care issues, for example. Forensic psychiatry does not aim to take on the totality of work concerned with difficult patients and medico-legal issues. Nevertheless, it is a resource which is readily available to other specialists, general practitioners, lawyers, police officers, probation officers, and others, when required.

Any professional who believes that he or she would be able to manage a case better with advice from a forensic psychiatry team should consider referring that case for advice. The advice might be about the management of difficult behaviour, about the range of services available for a particular patient, or the technical legal problems confronting the patient.

Forensic psychiatrists have access to treatment services which are not available in other subspecialties. For example, maximum security hospitals, medium security units, and prison units, are usually under the direction of forensic psychiatrists. Forensic psychiatrists are also fairly used to managing serious behavioural problems, particularly those which present long-term difficulties. They may, therefore, actively assist in the treatment of cases within the community. Sometimes this is done by the forensic team taking over the care of a difficult patient, sometimes it is done by joint working with regular advice being provided to the core workers. If there are specialized hostel facilities available to mentally disordered offenders of a particular dependent kind, then patients thought possibly suitable for such facilities should be referred to a forensic psychiatry team.

Advice about management, legal problems, services, and such like, can also be sought from forensic psychiatrists without a direct patient referral. In many places the writing of legal reports can be supervised by a forensic psychiatry consultant on request.

Epilepsy

Refer if there is:

- A major psychiatric disorder, particularly if it is due to or interacts with the epilepsy. This might include major affective disorder, psychosis, particularly schizophrenia-like psychosis of epilepsy or post-ictal psychosis, evidence of cognitive deterioration, more uncommonly, sexual disorders relating to seizure activity or to anticonvulsant treatment.

- Uncertainty about diagnosis especially if there is a possibility of pseudoseizures or if the seizure is thought to be due primarily to alcohol abuse.

- A strong psychological component. Seizure frequency is particularly influenced by stress. Some patients find it difficult to accept a diagnosis of epilepsy and this may influence treatment compliance.

Learning disability

Always refer when in doubt.

Refer before commencing any long-term drug therapy, particularly neuroleptics. Refer to access community support services. Do not refer simply as a means of disposal.

The elderly

Referral policies will vary from service to service. Commonly, old-age psychiatry services will be responsible for patients with mental disorders whose onset occurs after the age of 65 years. (In some services the age limit is 70 or even 75 years) Most old-age psychiatry services will take over the care of patients with pre-senile dementia (namely onset before 65 years of age) once the diagnosis has been made by general psychiatry or other medical services. Patients who have long-standing functional psychiatric illnesses who pass the age of 65 do *not* automatically transfer to old-age psychiatry. These patients generally remain the responsibility of general psychiatrists unless they develop a new mental disorder such as dementia.

Specialized psychotherapy

Psychotherapy can contribute usefully to patient care at two levels: case discussion and formal assessment. All patients, however they present, deserve consideration from a psychodynamic point of view, but not all would want or would be suitable for referral for assessment and treatment.

Case discussion

The best way to obtain a satisfactory service from psychotherapy is to keep a channel of communication open with the psychotherapist. An excellent way to do this is to have a regular case discussion seminar with the psychotherapist which all members of the multidisciplinary team may attend. Dynamic psychotherapists are as interested in the experience of working with the patient as in details of the history and presentation. Inevitably, those cases discussed will tend to be those who generate most emotion and controversy among those trying to help them. Commonly, such patients will tend to suffer from a personality disorder in addition to the 'Axis I' diagnosis. Case discussions help the staff keep track of countertransference interference with sound judgement and good management.

Referral for formal assessment

The main choice in referring an individual or a couple for psychological treatment is to decide between a psychodynamic assessment and a cognitive behavioural approach. Certain diagnostic categories invite the latter: for example, obsessive–compulsive disorder, specific phobias, agoraphobia, post-traumatic stress disorder, sexual dysfunction.

This approach is most suitable for patients who are motivated to be rid of their symptoms and who have little or no curiosity about their meaning or origin.

The more complicated the presenting clinical picture, especially by personality disorder or multiple symptoms, and the more obvious the patient's difficulties in the domain of personal relationships, the more likely it is that a combined or serial approach with psychodynamic psychotherapy may be necessary.

Psychodynamic assessment, as the first choice, is appropriate for any patient who can recognize their tendency to form the same dysfunctional relationships, who can see patterns in their life recurring, and who accepts responsibility for their difficulties, at least in so far as being motivated to seek a relationship within which to explore them.

Diagnostic categories are not so important, although patients commonly present in crisis with hypomania, depression, anxiety, somatic complaints, sexual deviations, conversion disorders, eating disorders, and relationship difficulties, or a combination of these. They frequently have some personality disorder. The focus of the psychodynamic assessment is the quality of the transference that develops, the nature of the defences mobilized against anxiety, and the patient's capacity to hear and make use of interpretations relating to these made by the psychotherapist.

As a general rule, it is helpful to wait until the immediate presenting crisis is resolved (by pharmacological first aid and supportive counselling) before it is possible to be sure that the patient is willing to undergo a psychotherapy assessment. It is most helpful to the psychotherapist that you do not pre-empt the outcome of the assessment by promising psychotherapy.

10
Early treatments

Acute psychosis

Advice on the managment of acute psychoses and on rapid tranquillization, are given in Figs. 10.1 and 10.2. Appendix 2 contains a list of antipsychotic drugs, and Appendix 3 a list of long-acting preparations. Information about clozapine will be found in Appendix 4, and equivalent doses of various neuroleptics in Appendix 5.

Rapid tranquillization

See Fig. 10.2.

Acute dystonia affecting respiration

Clinical features Abrupt onset, hours after commencing neuroleptic (often butyrophenone). Young > old. Painful muscular spasm with respiratory stridor and tongue protrusion, which induces panic.

Differential diagnosis Status epilepticus; trismus; foreign body obstruction; hysteria (rare).

Management Stop neuroleptic. Give IM antimuscarinic (procyclidine 5–10 mg). Reassure patient and staff. Check for cyanosis and administer oxygen, transfer to medical unit as required.

Neuroleptic malignant syndrome (NMS)

Neuroleptic malignant syndrome is a rare idiosyncratic reaction to neuroleptics characterized by: *intense extrapyramidal rigidity* and

Standard oral neuroleptic (e.g. chlorpromazine or haloperidol) at standard doses
Assess over at least 2–4 weeks

Ineffective ↓ Not tolerated

* Non-adherence is common, especially if patients do not collaborate in their choice of treatment

Effective → Tolerated

Continue with oral therapy or change to depot to assure adherence to therapy

---

Change to different class of oral neuroleptic at standard doses
Try sulpiride/risperidone if first drug poorly tolerated
Try risperidone if EPSE is severe or if negative symptoms predominate
Assess over at least 2–4 weeks

Ineffective ↓ Not tolerated

* Assess efficacy and tolerance with recognized rating scales e.g. BPRS, PANSS, ESRS, LUNSERS

* Avoid neuroleptic polypharmacy — oral + depot are rarely necessary

Effective → Tolerated

Continue with oral therapy or change to depot to assure adherence

---

Consider augmenting with lithium (if schizoaffective), benzodiazepines (to sedate), or carbamazepine (for aggression or as a mood stabilizer)
Assess over at least 2–4 weeks

Ineffective ↓ Not tolerated

Consider early use of short-term clonazepam if sedation is required in acute psychosis

Effective → Tolerated

Continue, but review need regularly. Long-term therapy with benzodiazepines not recommended

| If measured improvement, document in notes and continue, ? with depot. Review frequently |

Consider increasing dose of neuroleptic
May exceed BNF limits if Royal College guidelines followed — TPR/ECG, etc
(see BNF)
Assess over at least 2–4 weeks, but no longer than 3 months

Effective
→
Tolerated

Few data to support the use of high-dose neuroleptics

Ineffective ↓ Not tolerated

Change to clozapine
Give dose of 400 mg/day+
Assess over at least 6 months

Some support for the use of clozapine plasma levels — aim for a pre-dose level of 350 µg/L

| If measured improvement, continue at reduced dose |

Effective
→
Tolerated

Ineffective ↓ Not tolerated

Perform complete drug history
Review diagnosis
Consider withdrawing all (ineffective) drugs and give *most* effective drug previously prescribed at lowest dose

Fig. 10.1 Algorithm for the drug treatment of schizophrenia. EPSE, extrapyrimidal side-effects; BPRS, Brief Psychiatric Rating Scale; PANSS, Positive and negative symptom scale; ESRS, Extrapyramidal side effects rating scale; LUNSERS, Liverpool University side effect rating scale; BNF, British National Formulary; TPR, temperature, pulse, and respiration; ECG, electrocardiogram.

Notes: *
Seek advice from your consultant at any stage if you are in any doubt

Consider non-drug measures: talking-down, distraction, seclusion. Try oral therapy

Response → Consider starting/increasing regular oral medication

No response

* Monitor respiratory rate, pulse, BP, every 5 min
* Benzodiazepines safer than neuroleptics, but beware of accumulation. Use benzos alone if any cardiac disease.
* *Never* give Clopixol Acuphase to a struggling patient or to those who are neuroleptic naive.
* Procyclidine IV/IM must be available — ? give as prophylaxis

Give either:
haloperidol 5–10 mg IV + diazepam 10 mg IV
Wait ten minutes

or

droperidol 5–10mg IM + lorazepam 2 mg IM
Wait 30 minutes

Response → (Re)commence oral neuroleptics

or

Give zuclopenthixol acetate (Clopixol Acuphase) 50–150 mg. Peaks at 24–36 hours; effective for 72 hours

No response

(Continued)

* Facilities for mechanical ventilation/cardiac resus must be available
* If contact with patient is lost: monitor as for full anaesthetic procedure — use Pulse Oximeter
* Give flumazenil if respiratory rate drops below 10/minute
* Use IV route if IM is ineffective after three doses

* Do not use Amytal or paraldehyde without advice from consultant

* Actions in shaded boxes are for very exceptional circumstances

---

Repeat above
Wait 10 minutes for IV
or
30 minutes for IM
May repeat again
up to a maximum of 60 mg haloperidol + 60 mg diazepa,

No response

Seek advice from consultant/senior colleague

Advice to continue

Response

As above

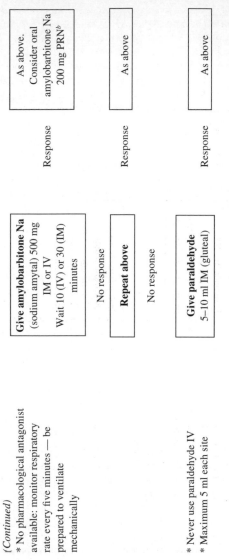

(Continued)

* No pharmacological antagonist available: monitor respiratory rate every five minutes — be prepared to ventilate mechanically

Give amylobarbitone Na (sodium amytal) 500 mg IM or IV

Wait 10 (IV) or 30 (IM) minutes

No response → **Repeat above**

No response →

As above. Consider oral amylobarbitone Na 200 mg PRN[b]

Response →

Response → As above

* Never use paraldehyde IV
* Maximum 5 ml each site

Give paraldehyde 5–10 ml IM (gluteal)

Response → As above

Fig. 10.2 Rapid tranquillization: algorithm for rapid control of the acutely disturbed patient. This algorithm is for guidance only: rigid adherence to it may not always be appropriate. Maximum rates of IV administration: amylobarbitone, 50 mg/min; diazepam, 5 mg/ml; droperidol, haloperidol, lorazepam: give over 2–3 min. **Never mix lorazepam or diazepam with other drugs in the same syringe. Never give diazepam IM.** PRN, as required.

other *dystonia; pyrexia* which may be mild; *autonomic dysfunction*; *sweating*; *clouding of consciousness*. There is substantial overlap with acute lethal catatonia. The incidence of the condition is variously reported as between 0.07 and 2 per cent, probably because of the lack of clear diagnostic criteria and the overlap with other severe extrapyramidal syndromes. Associated biochemical and other abnormalities include a grossly elevated *creatine phosphokinase, leucocytosis*, and a *raised erythrocyte sedimentation rate (ESR)*.

NMS has been reported with all neuroleptics and is unpredictable, although, in general, it is associated with larger doses of high-potency antipsychotics. This is not always the case. Its reported mortality varies between 12 and 18 per cent, usually as a consequence of autonomic instability (for example, cardiac arrest) or renal failure due to rhabdomyolysis and myoglobinuria.

Treatment of neuroleptic malignant syndrome (see schema, p. 188)

Ideally, all patients suspected of having NMS should be transferred to a medical intensive care facility. Immediate withdrawal of neuroleptics produces rapid resolution in early identified patients. A dopamine agonist, such as oral *bromocriptine* or *subcutaneous apomorphine*, is also recommended and sometimes *dantrolene*, as a peripheral muscle relaxant up to five times. Full medical supportive measures to maintain hydration, electrolyte status, and renal function should be available. In established cases these measures lead to a mean resolution time of 10 days

Treatment of the remaining psychiatric condition

ECT would appear to be the safest option. However, this should be deferred until after the episode since the anaesthetic risk is increased with autonomic dysfunction. A 'drug holiday' of 2 weeks is certainly recommended and diminishes the chance of recurrence on rechallenge. Treatment should be with ECT if ongoing psychiatric disturbance demands it. Ideally, rechallenge should be with a lower potency neuroleptic of a different chemical class. Patients need daily physical monitoring of blood pressure, consciousness, temperature, and creatinine phosphokinase (CPK) estimations during rechallenge. About one in six patients will suffer a recurrence after a rechallenge.

Algorithm for the treatment of neuroleptic malignant syndrome:

Transfer to acute medical ward or
ICU; monitor ECG, blood pressure, and
renal status
↓
Cessation of neuroleptics
↓
Bromocriptine 5–10 mg three time a day orally
(but if unable to swallow)
↓
Apomorphine infusion
subcutaneously 1 mg/h
↓
(no response)
↓
Dantrolene sodium
50 mg twice a day max. for 3 days

Acute mania and catatonia

Acute manic episodes are best treated with lithium. However, since it is difficult to administer an oral drug to an acute manic as well as make assessments for renal and thyroid function, it is often reserved as a prophylactic. Sedation in response to the behavioural disturbance is the usual aim. Butyrophenones are often the drug of choice, but there are few systematic clinical trials. Usually haloperidol or droperidol is used at doses of 10 mg 4 times a day. Sometimes benzodiazepines may be useful. Where lithium can be used it is better tolerated, has few extrapyramidal effects, and is non-sedating.

Most psychiatrists recommend that higher doses of lithium are used to give a level of about 1 mmol/litre. Careful monitoring for side-effects is recommended at these higher doses. In severely disturbed patients, patients refusing medication, or in a manic emergency, ECT is recommended. This should be bilateral because of the need for a rapid response. The disturbance usually abates after one or two applications. However, it is recommended that a full course of 8–12 applications be pursued.

Catatonia is now rarely seen in developed countries. The most important principle in treating catatonia is in the differential diagnosis to distinguish it from NMS and manic or depressive stupor (see p. 114). Catatonia, in acute schizophrenia, may be characterized by waxy flexibility, negativism, automatic obedience, and a 'wooden' affect. Treatment of the catatonia is of the underlying condition. However, in persistent or distressing states, benzodiazepines or ECT may be tried.

Severe depression

Levels of in-patient supervision for a suicidal patient

When a suicidal patient is admitted, the admitting doctor should discuss the level of supervision with a senior nurse. The options are:

- *Close observation.* Here the patient is always in sight of the supervising nurse. This is the normal practice when a depressed patient is admitted with high-suicide risk. Usually the risk abates within a few days, but the level of risk needs to be assessed daily.

- *Continuous supervision.* Here the patient is always within reach of a nurse. This is used when the patient is at immediate risk from self-destructive, including bulimic, behaviour.

- *Routine nursing care.*

Assessment of other physical risks

Weight loss is common and, unless severe, is not a cause for concern, but dehydration is always an indication for admission and institution of a fluid balance chart with assessment of electrolytes. Skilled nursing persuades many patients to correct dehydration, but if this fails then other action is needed, including intravenous rehydration and emergency ECT.

Electroconvulsive therapy

Indications

Depressive illnesses

ECT is an effective antidepressant for depressive illnesses regardless of subtype. The best predictor of response to ECT is the presence and number of typical symptoms and signs of depression. It is particularly useful when symptoms include psychomotor retardation, psychotic features such as delusions and/or hallucinations, and can be life-saving if the patient is suicidal or fails to maintain an adequate nutritional or hydration status.

There is no justification in reserving ECT as a treatment of 'last resort'. Indications for its use as a primary treatment include patient preference, a past history of response to ECT, a history of poor drug response (such as non-compliance or intolerable or potentially severe side-effects), the need for a rapid response to treatment, and if the risks of other treatments exceed those for ECT.

Manic illness

ECT has been less frequently used for mania since the advent of lithium and neuroleptics, but it remains an effective treatment. Indications for its use include the need for a speedy therapeutic response, as a safe alternative to high-dose medications, if patients have drug-resistant mania, or have 'rapid cycling' mania.

Schizophrenia

ECT may be effective in patients with Type 1 schizophrenia, particularly when psychotic symptoms are associated with affective symptoms and/or abnormal motor activity such as catatonic excitement or immobility. It may be used if the patient needs a speedy response, is unable to tolerate medications, or has failed to respond to an adequate dose of neuroleptics. It is not recommended for Type 2 schizophrenia in the absence of an affective component.

Other conditions

ECT may be effective in the post-partum psychoses and catatonia. It has also been used in resistant epilepsy and Parkinson's disease (particularly those with the 'on–off' phenomenon: alternating periods of akinetic rigidity and hyperkinesia).

Contraindications

Although there are no 'absolute' contraindications to ECT, co-existing medical problems must be treated and physical health optimized. Pregnancy and old age are not contraindications to ECT. 'High-risk' cases, such as patients with a recent myocardial infarction, cerebrovascular accident, or raised intracranial pressure must be assessed on an individual basis with respect to the risk/benefit of ECT. Close liaison between the psychiatrist, anaesthetist, and physician is essential in such cases.

Side-effects

The mortality associated with ECT is approximately 2 per 100 000 treatments, a figure similar to that for minor surgical procedures. The most common side-effects include headache, memory impairment, and confusion. Rarer side-effects include prolonged seizures, tardive seizures, manic rebound, and physical complications such as ruptured bladder or aspiration pneumonia. Modification of anaesthesia with a barbiturate anaesthetic and muscle relaxant have decreased morbidity as have improvements in ECT monitoring. While bilateral application of ECT is the recommended means of inducing a seizure, the use of unilateral non-dominant ECT can be used if cognitive side-effects are troublesome.

Preparation

A full physical examination and detailed medical history are mandatory in all patients. It is suggested that patients be given a baseline full blood count and urea and electrolyte levels measured. The anaesthetist should be informed when ECT is being arranged and any problems should be noted and addressed in advance. As for any general anaesthetic, the patient should fast for at least 6 hours and dentures be removed.

A pre-ECT nursing checklist should accompany the patient. The ECT treatment and prescription form should document the physical health, indications for ECT, the relevant past medical and psychiatric history, past treatments, present and recently discontinued medications, the legal status, and the consultant's prescription. A fully informed consent must be obtained or the relevant legal documents pertinent to the administration of ECT.

Administration

The ECT machine in use should be safe, easy to use, with a wide range of output and stimulus parameters. Further reading is recommended regarding initial dosage and titration of stimulus. A therapeutic seizure should be bilateral and of approximately 15 seconds duration when measured visually, and approximately 20–50 seconds on the EEG if available. The number and frequency of treatments is determined by clinical progress, as is the end-point. A common policy is twice weekly administration for 6–12 treatments.

Deliberate self-harm (DSH)

Assess the patient's mental state in the light of the social environment and coping skills:

- Treatment of physical condition in DSH patients takes precedence (cave: long-term effects of paracetamol).
- Suicide and repetition risk cannot be assessed in drowsy patients.

- Patients with low repetition risk and no mental illness. Principles of *crisis intervention* apply: 'understand' attempt; mobilize resources; consider a 'non-DSH' contract; discharge preferably to relatives; inform GP; appointment with DSH-liaison or alcohol/drugs services team.

- Most high-risk patients will be mentally ill. Management depends on community resources (supportive relatives, GP, community psychiatric nurse (CPN)). In case of unacceptable risk consider admission, compulsorily if necessary.

- For frequent repeaters the same principles apply; a long-term management plan is vital to avoid counterproductive admissions.

- Risk can never be excluded completely, adequacy of note-taking and interdisciplinary communication vital.

Overdoses

Opiates

This causes varying degrees of coma, respiratory depression, and pinpoint pupils. The short-acting opiate antagonist naloxone is indicated if there is coma or bradypnoea. Dosage is 0.8–2 mg repeated at intervals of 2–3 minutes to a maximum of 10 mg if respiratory function does not improve. It is available in preloaded syringes. Due to its short action it may be necessary to set up a naloxone infusion which is adjusted according to response. This may occur in patients who have overdosed on methadone — methadone has a long half-life. In severe cases mechanical ventilation may be necessary.

Following the administration of naloxone a patient will experience acute withdrawal. It is important to continue to observe them for 24 hours, but, commonly, craving for drugs will lead them to discharge themselves.

Methadone

If a methadone overdose is reported, but there are, as yet, no signs of respiratory depression, activated charcoal should be given and the patient observed closely. Inducing patients to vomit is not recommended because of the risk of the rapid onset of CNS depression and unconsciousness which could lead to choking.

Cocaine

Cocaine overdose is characterized by cardiovascular complications including arrhythmias, cardiac ischaemia, myocarditis, cardiomyopathy, and hypertension. Seizures and hyperpyrexias also occur. Treatment is supportive and patients need medical help as soon as possible.

Alcohol dependence

The alcohol withdrawal syndrome

Individuals will only experience symptoms of alcohol withdrawal if they are physically dependent on alcohol. Thus some heavy drinkers experience no withdrawal symptoms, whereas others show evidence of mild or moderate withdrawal, and a few will develop a life-threatening disturbance.

Symptoms of alcohol withdrawal start approximately 3–6 hours after the last drink. Early symptoms include tremor, sweats, nausea, insomnia, and anxiety. Transient auditory hallucinations in clear consciousness may occur. There is a risk of alcohol withdrawal seizures between 10 and 60 hours; these generalized (grand mal) seizures are often associated with hypoglycaemia, hypokalaemia, hypomagnesaemia, and concurrent epilepsy. Most alcohol withdrawal syndromes resolve within 72 hours of drinking cessation. The more severe the withdrawal, the longer the duration of symptoms. A few patients go on to develop delirium tremens (DTs) around 72 hours after the last drink. Symptoms include severe clouding of consciousness, confusion, hallucinations in any modality, tremor, fear, paranoid delusions, restlessness, and agitation. The condition usually lasts for 3–5 days, with gradual resolution. Predisposing factors include hypoglycaemia, hypokalaemia, hypocalcaemia, and intercurrent infection.

A few patients with thiamine deficiency may develop Wernicke's encephalopathy, and not all will show the classic triad of ataxia, ophthalmoplegia, and abnormal mental state.

Delirium tremens and Wernicke's encephalopathy are medical emergencies requiring immediate hospital admission.

Treatment of alcohol withdrawal

Most patients can be detoxified safely and effectively in the community. Indications for in-patient detoxification include severe dependence, a history of delirium tremens or alcohol withdrawal seizures, coexistent medical problems, an unsupportive home environment, and a previously failed community detoxification programme. All patients need general support and a proportion will need pharmacotherapy for the withdrawal symptoms. Benzodiazepines are the treatment of choice, and individual doctors should become familiar with one drug of this class. Because of the great range in the severity of the alcohol withdrawal syndrome, a range of drug doses is indicated. A mild to moderate withdrawal syndrome in an out-patient should respond to chlordiazepoxide (Librium) 5–10 mg three or four times daily. A moderate withdrawal syndrome may require a dose in the order of 15–20 mg three or four times daily. Community and out-patient detoxifications should last approximately one week. Higher doses are required in the in-patient setting, for example chlordiazepoxide 40–60 mg three or four times a day, reducing over 7–10 days. Chlormethiazole (Heminevrin) may still have a role in the in-patient setting, but is contraindicated for community detoxification.

Appropriate use of benzodiazepines should prevent the development of alcohol withdrawal seizures, thus anticonvulsants are not indicated routinely. However, carbamazepine may be considered if there is a history of seizures during any previous withdrawal episodes, or a history of untreated epilepsy.

Because of the risk of a Wernicke's encephalopathy in these patients, prophylactic thiamine (vitamin B) supplementation is recommended. Thiamine may be taken orally, but absorption is poor. In the case of confirmed or imminent acute Wernicke's encephalopathy parenteral administration (intramuscular or slow intravenous) of high-potency B vitamins is indicated once or twice daily for 3–5 days. Caution is needed because of the risk of a serious allergic reaction.

Delirium tremens

Clinical features

Alcohol withdrawal phenomena. Rapid onset of hallucinations, fear, disorientation and confusion, tremor, tachycardia, fever, overactivity, and clamminess occur.

Differential diagnosis

Delirium due to another cause.

Management

Full blown syndrome should be managed on medical unit (mortality >5 per cent). Give adequate sedation (chlordiazepoxide 40 mg 4 times daily.) and fluid replacement. Administer thiamine as prophylaxis against Wernicke's encephalopathy. Beware withdrawal seizures.

Wernicke's encephalopathy

Clinical features

Acute onset of nystagmus, gaze palsies, gait ataxia and confusional state due to thiamine deficiency are most commonly seen in alcoholics, but also may occur in malnutrition and prolonged vomiting (and therefore should be considered in patients with eating disorders).

Differential diagnosis

Infective or metabolic encephalopathy, hydrocephalus, tumour, posterior circulation infarction or haemorrage.

Management

Thiamine should be given as soon as the diagnosis is entertained, preferably intravenously. Full recovery is possible with rapid treatment; however, many go on to develop a chronic Korsakoff's psychosis.

Drug misuse

Basic management

- A knowledge of local patterns of drug use, practicalities of drug use, and terms used can be important in establishing rapport.
- A non-judgemental attitude is essential, both with regard to drug use and associated activity such as sex and work.
- Consistency of communication between different staff members is important to minimize the potential for confused messages.
- Be clear about what the patient can expect in the way of treatment in your particular setting.
- Be clear about what is expected of the patient in your treatment setting.
- Your contact with a drug user may be the only one they have with services for some time, especially if it takes place in an emergency setting. Emphasizing general health care needs, education, and harm reduction advice is important in this situation (pp. 204–5).
- A change in drug use in established misusers usually takes place through several cyles of contemplation, change and relapse. Avoid the disappointment which can result from the expectation of sudden lasting change, but maintain hope and optimism in your attitude!

Opiates

Opiate withdrawal

Symptoms of withdrawal from heroin can be expected to start within 12 hours of the last dose of the drug. They peak within

72 hours and are likely to be essentially over within a week, although milder symptoms and sleep difficulty can persist for several weeks. Patients met in clinical practice are also likely to be withdrawing from methadone which has a longer half-life and, therefore, a withdrawal syndrome which is delayed in onset (usually at least 24 hours after last dose), peaks after several days, and is likely to last longer than a week. The pattern of withdrawal from other opiates which may be encountered can be predicted from the half-life and dose. Withdrawal from partial opiate agonists (for example, buprenorphine) is typically described as milder than that from full agonists.

Withdrawal from opiates is due to unopposed activity by neurotransmitter systems which have adapted to the presence of opiates. The symptoms can be predicted from consideration of the effects of unopposed high levels of activity in the locus coeruleus (central noradrenergic) and peripheral sympathetic autonomic activity. Hence:

- pupillary dilation
- rhinorrhoea
- lacrimation
- sneezing
- piloerection
- nausea
- vomiting

- abdominal cramp
- diarrhoea
- skeletal muscle cramp
- anxiety
- dysphoria
- tachycardia
- elevated blood pressure.

Also likely to be present are a craving for opiates and opiate-seeking behaviour.

Withdrawal of opiates can reveal masked underlying symptoms such as pain. Although markedly unpleasant, the withdrawal syndrome is not directly physically dangerous. Although it may be expected to vary with the dose of opiate, the severity of opiate withdrawal syndrome is also markedly susceptible to other factors such as the physical and social environment.

Symptomatic relief with non-opiate medication
This is an option which can be offered by any doctor when a patient presents in withdrawal. Medication to consider includes:

- metaclopramide
- diphenoxylate + atropine (Lomotil)
- mebeverine.

Prescribe the above in normal doses for the duration of the withdrawal period. Diazepam may also be appropriate in this situation to help sleep, muscle spasm, and anxiety. However, it should only be prescribed when there is no suspicion of benzodiazepine misuse by the patient, in moderate doses, and strictly for the duration of the expected withdrawal period only.

Methadone
Methadone is commonly used to assist withdrawal from opiates. Initially, the patient should be stabilized on a dose of methadone sufficient to control withdrawal symptoms. The dose of methadone is then tapered according to an exponential decay curve (that is to say, larger decrements initially). In practice, the time over which this is done varies with the situation, from reduction over 10 days in inpatient settings to much slower reduction in out-patients. Overall benefit is probably greatest if the reduction regime proceeds flexibly as planned with the patient rather than rigidly according to a protocol.

Lofexidine
Lofexidine is a centrally acting alpha-$_2$ agonist and is effective in reducing withdrawal symptoms. Clinical evaluation on in-patient units and in out-patient settings in the UK is at an early stage. It has the advantage of causing less hypotension than clonidine (another centrally acting alpha-$_2$ agonist which has been used for some time in in-patient settings).

Opiates — basic substitute prescribing

Methadone is a synthetic long-acting opiate which may be taken by mouth. Substitute prescribing of methadone for heroin provides opportunities for several types of treatment, rarely:

- Short-term detoxification.
- Long-term [months] out-patient effort to achieve abstinence.
- Maintenance treatment.

The aim of maintenance treatment does not include abstinence except in the much longer term (years). Treatment aims of maintenance are the reduction in frequency of injecting, reduction in amount of illicit drug use, reduction in crime, and social and psychological stabilization.

There are several issues which are common to all methadone prescribing. Prior to starting it should be established that the patient is already opiate dependent. Methods include:

- history-taking
- detection of heroin in several urine samples
- inspection of injection sites in an intravenous user
- observation of withdrawal symptoms.

The initial methadone dose can be estimated from the history of heroin consumption, but it is usual to start with a safe dose (20 mg in adults) administered in a setting where the response can be assessed later that same day or the following day, and gradually titrating the dose up to the desired dose. In a situation aimed at detoxification the dose will be the lowest which controls withdrawal symptoms, but it may be considerably higher when maintenance is the aim since higher doses are associated with better outcomes.

Methadone is prescribed from a hospital on a pink prescription which allows for multiple dispensing dates. It should usually be prescribed for dispensing on a daily basis. The prescription needs to specify the type of methadone, daily dose, and total amount in words and figures, frequency of dispensing, and start date. for example:

Oral methadone liquid 1 mg/ml 40 mg (forty) daily for 14 days. Dispense daily, but for two days on Saturdays. Start on 1st July 1998. Total dose 560 mg (five hundred and sixty).

The conditions on which the prescription is offered should be clearly agreed upon between the patient and the prescriber before commencing a prescription. Issues to be agreed include: the length of prescription; frequency with which the prescriber will see the patient; lack of acceptability of aggression, threats, or actual violence; alcohol consumption; urine testing in which heroin and methadone use can be distinguished and whether continued evidence of illicit drug use is acceptable; other treatment to be offered in addition to prescribing. It is also good practice also to identify at the outset those targets which, it is anticipated, the patient will be helped to achieve with the treatment offered, and future dates at which the treatment will be reviewed.

Benzodiazepines

Benzodiazepine withdrawal

The benzodiazepine group of drugs also contains drugs with a wide range of half-lives which affect the pattern and severity of withdrawal syndrome. Examples are:

Short-acting	Intermediate	Long-acting:
• triazolam	• oxazepam	• diazepam
• temazepam	• nitrazepam	• flunitrazepam

The onset of symptoms may be rapid. Triazolam was reported to result in rebound wakefulness and withdrawal within the course of a single night, this resulted in its withdrawal from the UK market. In clinical practice with the street drug-using population, the most likely benzodiazepines to be encountered are temazepam and diazepam. Often the use will be a mixture of drugs including these two. Withdrawal symptoms will have an insidious onset in this situation and may occur days after the last dose of diazepam. Symptoms are due to unopposed activity of the gamma-aminobutyric acid (GABA) complex.

They consist of general symptoms of anxiety:

- tremor
- tachycardia
- tachypnoea
- nausea

- abdominal cramp
- skeletal muscle cramp
- diarrhoea
- psychic anxiety;

and, in addition:

- seizures
- perceptual distortion.

The symptoms can be more subtle and difficult to distinguish from differential diagnoses, such as anxiety disorders, than opiate withdrawal. However, benzodiazepine withdrawal carries a greater physical danger because of the risk of seizures.

Stabilization on to diazepam and gradual tapering of the dose will control withdrawal symptoms. As with opiates, the time over which the tapering occurs is shorter and more rigidly determined in in-patients (10–21 days). Reduction in out-patients is more likely to take place over the course of several weeks and to involve the patient in determining the rate of reduction (see below).

In patients with an established history of seizures a covering dose of an antiepileptic, such as carbamazepine, may aid a planned detoxification programme.

Benzodiazepines — basic substitute prescribing

Diazepam is usually chosen as a substitute for illicit diazepam, temazepam, and other benzodiazepines. This is primarily due to its long half-life. The evidence for its success in substitute prescribing, in those who are usually poly-drug misusers, is much more controversial than that of methadone for heroin. For example, in many cases there is no obvious benefit in terms of changed injecting practice. It is harder to be clear in follow-up whether the patient is being compliant since urine testing provides no useful evidence to back-up clinical history and examination. In practice, decisions are made according to local practice, local population of drug misusers, and individual clinical assessment.

A starting dose of diazepam is negotiated which will prevent withdrawal, and a reduction regime agreed with the patient before starting the prescription. The agreement may set out a rigid structure or may simply be the boundaries within which change will be negotiated as the treatment progresses. Most benzodiazepines are prescribed with abstinence as a goal, at least within a few months, but there are some individuals for whom a period of maintenance is agreed. Diazepam currently can be prescribed only on yellow single dispensing prescriptions. Arranging daily dispensing, although desirable in many cases, has considerable implications in terms of inconvenience. As with methadone, agreement of the conditions of treatment, criteria for review, and frequency of review, must be clear at the outset.

Amphetamines, cocaine, and other stimulant drugs

Stimulant drugs such as amphetamaines, cocaine, and 'ecstasy' do not produce a major physical withdrawal syndrome and can be stopped abruptly. Many stimulant users who are psychologically dependent experience insomnia and depressed mood when the drug is stopped. Antidepressants such as desipramine may be helpful, but many stimulant users just need advice regarding the likely symptoms, reassurance that they will pass, and a safe place to get through this period. Some patients may become acutely suicidal and will require hospital admission and close observation.

Substitute prescribing of stimulant drugs is rarely recommended and should be left for specialist treatment services. However, remember that stimulant drugs, like opiates, may be injected and advice on harm reduction may be appropriate (see p. 204).

Stimulant-induced confusion and anxiety states

Cocaine and other stimulants such as ecstasy (Methylene dioxy Methamphetamine; MDMA) and amphetamines can cause acute effects which can sometimes be severe enough to present to the general psychiatrist. These states are commonly of euphoria or anxiety, but may proceed to more severe symptoms such as paranoid ideation leading to vigilant and aggressive behaviour and auditory or visual hallucinations. Insight is usually retained or only transiently impaired. Management involves calming and reassuring the patient until the effects wear off. Occasionally oral diazepam (10–20 mg) may be needed and in severe cases antipsychotic medication. If symptoms persist a drug-induced psychosis may result requiring general psychiatric management.

Hallucinogenic drugs

Hallucinogenic drugs such as LSD do not produce a physical withdrawal syndrome and can be stopped abruptly. There is no role for substitute prescribing. However, some people experience severe psychological distress during or after using hallucinogens and may need symptomatic treatment (such as a brief course of benzodiazepines to reduce anxiety), and a safe place to be while the experience passes.

Harm reduction

This is an approach to the management of drug users which was developed following the discovery of HIV in the intravenous drug-using population. The transmission of blood-borne viruses may be one of many possible harms resulting from drug use. The approach assumes that reducing the harm from the use of drugs may take priority over the reduction of drug use itself. It assumes a hierarchy of treatment goals with abstinence being the ideal outcome, but with intermediate goals achievable. For instance, an objective may be to reduce intravenous drug use and transfer to oral drug use or to move from risky injecting where needles are being shared to safer injecting using clean injecting equipment.

Basic harm reduction advice should be available whenever a drug user presents to a service and should include education about the following:

- Advice on safe injecting techniques. This will include information on not sharing or reusing needles, skin cleaning, and the danger of some injecting sites — groin and femoral particularly.

- Advice on how to obtain clean injecting equipment. This will depend on the area, but may be from a local drugs agency or a pharmacy needle-exchange scheme.

- Advice on safer sex. This will include advice on how the virus is transmitted sexually — by vaginal or anal intercourse and less frequently by oral sex — and on the correct use of condoms.

- Advice on how to clean injecting equipment if it must be reused. This is achieved using ordinary domestic bleach followed by at least three rinses with clean cold water.

- Advice on the dangers of overdose from opiates. This includes an awareness of problems with losing tolerance after a period of lower drug intake, such as in prison, and the dangers of new supplies of a drug which may be of higher purity.

- Advice on the dangers of prescribed and non-prescribed drugs to children. Methadone overdoses in children are common and any amount may be dangerous and need hospital treatment.

Other harm reduction interventions for drug users would include:

- hepatitis B immunization for non-immune individuals;
- HIV and hepatitis testing with appropriate pre- and post-test counselling;
- prescription of oral substitute drugs (see pp. 199 and 202).

Somatization

Immediate management

Management has several strands. First, to engage the patient in some form of dialogue. Second, to reduce further doctor visits, investigations, and so on. Third, if possible, to treat any underlying psychological disorder. It is essential that the patient feels understood — listen to the whole history of the symptoms and its impact. You are not taking a history in order to diagnose ischaemic heart disease, but so that the patient feels you have listened and understood their predicament and suffering. See the patient regularly, but not in response to symptoms. Do not say: 'Come and see me when you feel bad', but: 'Come every month anyway'. In a session you will usually have to listen to some account of the symptoms and their impact, even if you can do nothing about them. It can be useful to split the session in two — spend the first 15 minutes talking about symptoms and health, and then say: 'Now let's use the time for something else', and allow the patient to set another agenda.

More specific techniques, usually following cognitive behavioural principles, have been found successful. These usually involve some combination of cognitive work, looking at explanations for symptoms, generating alternative explanations, and looking at the links between sleep, mood, illness fears, and symptoms. This may be followed by some form of activity management programme with the intention of reducing the link between the experience of symptoms and some maladaptive behaviour pattern (such as going to bed). It is useful to be able to give sensible explanations for symptoms so that patients: (1) have an understanding of why they experience symptoms and (2) do not feel that you believe their symptoms are imaginary. Explaining the role of muscle tension in headache or chest pain, anxiety in palpitations, poor sleep and daytime fatigue, inactivity in muscle pain, and hyperventilation in chest pain can all be useful.

Symptom checklists can be useful — partly to monitor progress and particularly if planning an intervention (such as antidepressants) in order to check that any reported side-effects really are new. The underlying principle is to enable the patient to take over responsibility for their illness and recovery (and not rely on doctors, drugs, surgical procedures, and so on), but without feeling any guilt or blame for getting ill in the first place. This is harder than it sounds.

Things not to do

If the patient has a specific illness belief ('candida', 'ME', 'chronic allergy') do not question this, even if there is no corroborating medical evidence. Never get into a confrontation, or say: 'This illness doesn't exist'. Instead, having accepted the label, move on to: 'How can we help you live with the symptoms/ distress' or: 'How can we help you reduce your pain/disability, etc?' Never attempt to switch the patient from a solely physical to a solely psychological model. This is both inappropriate and largely impossible. Having obtained a full history, and made certain that basic investigations have been performed — such as thyroid function tests (TFTs) and/or ESR — do not refer to more specialists or perform more tests, unless some new indication comes along suggestive of a different problem.

Pharmacological management

Not often helpful. However, antidepressants can be effective. Contrary to conventional psychiatric teaching, there is some evidence that low-dose tricyclics can be effective for problems such as pain and sleep disorder. Many patients will be reluctant to take antidepressants, but may accept them on that basis.

Response to treatment

Most patients with somatization are seen in primary care, and usually are easy to engage and they respond well to simple treatments. Cognitive behavioural treatments are successful in those with discrete disorders such as atypical chest pain, low back pain, or chronic fatigue. However, those with long illness histories, who may fulfill criteria for somatization disorder, have a poor prognosis. 'Damage limitation', long-term support, and encouragement may be indicated.

Sexual disorders

Sexual dysfunctions

Management

General management is best undertaken with both partners (if available) and will include both sexual homework exercises and couple relationship work. If there is no partner, or the partner is unavailable, it is still possible to treat the individual, but modifications have to be made to the approach and the prognosis is more uncertain.

Behavioural approaches
The sensate focus technique of Masters and Johnson is widely used as a basic form of 'homework exercise' in most sex therapy. There is a ban on intercourse, and instead a form of prolonged foreplay is designed to improve communication on sexual matters and to reduce performance anxiety. The couple then progress to genital contact and to specific techniques for each specific dysfunction. For *premature ejaculation* the Semans' stop–start technique is used, stimulating the erect penis and stopping at the 'point of inevitability' just before ejaculation. For *delayed ejaculation* the technique of penile 'superstimulation' is recommended, perhaps with the aid of a vibrator, and this is usually more successful if the man can already ejaculate in masturbation rather than if he has a total inability to ejaculate. For *erectile dysfunction* gradual progression from sensate focus to penetration in the 'woman above'

position is recommended, with a progression to physical or pharmacological approaches if necessary (see below). For *anorgasmia* the couple are asked to practice clitoral stimulation, including the use of vibrators. For *vaginismus* the use of finger dilatation or of graduated dilators is recommended, followed by a careful progression to intercourse. For *dyspareunia* the treatment depends on the cause, and gynaecological procedures may be needed. In those without a physical cause, sensate focus, relaxation, different positions for intercourse, and relationship therapy may be useful. For *disorders of sexual desire* the approach is more variable, depending on the factors contributing to it: it may include couple relationship therapy, individual psychotherapy, post-traumatic counselling, antidepressant treatment, hormone therapy, advice on lifestyle changes, and other measures.

Psychotherapeutic approaches
Psychodynamic therapy is used for the individual with a dysfunction, especially when a 'block' is reached and progress ceases. Short-term dynamic therapy may be used in the course of sex therapy, and longer term therapy may be given in addition if other indications are present.

Cognitive therapy may be used in cases where there is depression or anxiety to be treated. In those with post-traumatic states (for example, following rape or sexual abuse) specific post-traumatic counselling may be given.

Relationship therapy
This is indicated in most cases of dysfunction in couples, especially if there are resentments or tensions present. Couple therapy may be psychodynamic, behavioural, cognitive, or systemic, or combinations of these (see p. 213). Relationship therapy is very useful in couples in which one partner is more enthusiastic than the other for sex (disorders of desire).

Mechanical or pharmacological treatment
Used mainly in *erectile dysfunction*. Penile rings and vacuum pumps can improve erections, and are acceptable to many couples. Yohimbine by mouth can improve the quality of erection as well as increasing sexual drive, but is not fully approved by the

Committee on the Safety of Medicines. Intracavernosal injections of prostaglandin or papaverine reliably produce erections, but are less acceptable to some couples as a means of allowing intercourse. If the cavernosal blood supply is shown to be inadequate (by arteriograms), surgery may be attempted to increase the arterial input; if the venous drainage can be shown to be excessive (through abnormal veins or fistulae, as shown in cavernosograms) surgical ligature of the veins may be tried. Neither of these surgical procedures is guaranteed to be successful. In extreme cases where no other method has succeeded it is possible to replace the corpora cavernosa with either semi-flexible Teflon rods or inflatable hollow tubes: these methods are successful in many cases, but late failures can occur, and the loss of natural function is, of course, irreversible after such an operation. In *premature ejaculation* it is possible to achieve some delay by utilizing a side-effect of the SSRI drugs or clomipramine. The effect is not however predictable, and is often quite small.

Vibrators are used in *female anorgasmia* and in *delayed ejaculation* in males, with variable success. Hormone replacement in post-menopausal women can reverse *atrophic vaginitis*, a frequent cause of pain and bleeding on intercourse. Hormone replacement in men is not as widely accepted, and should be reserved for cases with demonstrated androgen deficiency.

Course of sexual dysfunctions

The course of these conditions is very variable. It should be emphasized that, in most cases, 'cure' is not to be expected, but considerable improvement can follow a course of treatment.

Erectile dysfunction
This can be reversed in the great majority of men by one or other of the available treatments.

Premature ejaculation
Although it can be considerably improved, complete resolution is unusual. A combination of the stop–start technique with medication is probably the best approach for intractable cases, and results in adequate control in many.

Delayed ejaculation

Delayed ejaculation can be treated more successfully if it is 'situational' (that is to say, restricted to intercourse rather than present in all sexual activity); even in these cases, however there are some who fail to improve sufficiently, and if fertility is the issue the couple may have to resort to assisted fertilization.

Vaginismus

This has a better prognosis than many dysfunctions. If the couple achieve intercourse as a result of therapy (and this depends on the male as well as the female partner co-operating with treatment) it is unusual to see relapse, except perhaps transiently after childbirth.

Female anorgasmia

The absence of orgasm is relatively easy to treat, but the couple should be reminded that it is easier for most women to climax during clitoral stimulation, including the use of vibrators, than in intercourse, so the goals of therapy may have to be modified to help the couple incorporate clitoral stimulation into their activities.

Dyspareunia

Here the prognosis depends on its cause, and in many cases this is in the gynaecological rather than the psychological field. Where there is no physical cause the prognosis after treatment is reasonably good.

Loss of sexual desire

In both in men and women this has a very variable prognosis, according to the predisposing and precipitating factors. Where it appears to be a matter for negotiation between partners to achieve a more acceptable balance the outlook is often good; where it is associated with depression it depends on the treatment of the depression; where there are early traumatic experiences or other individual causes the outlook is more variable, and depends on the management of the other problems.

Sexual deviations and gender dysphoria

Management

If the deviation is harmful it is usual for the police and the courts to be involved before psychiatrists. Some patients, however, come to psychiatrists first, and then ethical dilemmas can arise over disclosure. The general rule is that if there is criminal activity taking place, especially if it involves a child, the doctor is bound to break the usual rules of confidentiality and inform the social services and/or police as what has been disclosed.

Management of any deviation is much easier and treatment more likely to be successful if the patient is either self-referred or comes with a clear aim of reducing the deviant behaviour. Those who are referred by courts or come as a result of pressure from family members or advisers are much less likely to do well.

Treatment is by behavioural, cognitive, or dynamic psychotherapy, by couple or family therapy, or by medication.

Behavioural and cognitive

Orgasmic conditioning is a relatively weak form of treatment, but may be useful in those deviants who have an alternative outlet for their sexuality. Aversion therapy, usually self-aversion using elastic bands round the wrist, is a fairly useful method for reducing unwanted sexual drives. Covert sensitization, using aversive cognitions as the negative consequence, is more acceptable to many patients and may be as effective as aversion. Both may be incorporated into various self-control packages to be applied when the patient is in danger of expressing his deviance, and, in addition, other cognitive techniques such as increased victim empathy and 'walking away' can be used in well-motivated patients. Many of these forms of treatment for deviation are used in group therapy, which may be given in specialized clinics or in probation settings.

Psychodynamic therapy

This is given in various specialized clinics, and is aimed at the underlying conflict rather than the deviant behaviour itself. It is probably most useful where (as often happens) the patient has experienced abusive relationships in the past.

Couple therapy

In some milder cases where the couple has a conflict over unusual sexual activities it is possible to help them to adjust to the deviant behaviour within the relationship, for example by incorporating the activity into their normal sexual life.

Family therapy

In some families in which there has been incestuous sexual abuse it is possible to rehabilitate the family (normally after a court hearing) using family therapy to enable then to live together. This is, however, quite rare, and depends on good motivation and general relationships within the family, as well as full social work support for the child.

Medication

In cases where the patient wishes to be free of all sexual urges the use of antilibidinal medication can be considered. Cyproterone acetate is the most satisfactory, but ethinyloestradiol and medroxyprogesterone may be used as alternatives. Ethical questions may be raised, especially in younger patients.

Course

This is very variable, depending on the type of deviation, but in very few cases can it be stated that the patient is 'cured' after treatment. It is much more a question of achieving better control of the behaviour. In some cases the behaviour is mild and not dangerous, and control makes it possible to lead a normal life, but in others custodial sentencing is the only way to protect society.

Transsexualism

It is important not to move too quickly into gender reassignment procedures, and it is usual to recommend that the patient should live as a member of the opposite sex for a period of two years, usually with the aid of hormone therapy, before the consideration of any surgery. It is then possible, in selected cases, to carry out gender reassignment operations with hormone therapy. However, a good deal of counselling is necessary after surgery, and adjustment is variable.

Couple and relationship problems

Management

This will vary according to the type of therapy involved.

Psychodynamic approach
Here the emphasis is on increasing the couple's understanding of underlying conflicts and unrealistic expectations, and interpretation of the transference to the therapist(s) is one of the methods used to achieve this. Therapy is relatively slow and long term.

Behavioural approaches
These involve the use of a more direct, short term, problem-solving method with an emphasis on negotiating differences, planning strategies for future avoidance of problems, and improving the clarity of communication.

Systemic couple approach
This therapy is more interested in helping the couple to change their interaction in terms of boundaries, power differences, closeness and distance, commitment and exclusiveness, and the eradication of symptoms since they are no longer necessary to 'stabilize the system'.

Mixed or combination approaches
There are many such approaches to treatment, for example psychodynamic-behavioural therapy, behavioural-systems therapy, and 'intersystem' therapy.

Course

The results of couple therapy may be evaluated in terms of improvement in the relationship, reduction of symptoms, prevention of divorce, or the continued welfare of children. No method is invariably better than another, but behavioural methods have been more frequently evaluated and usually shown to be effective. However, other methods, when compared to behavioural ones, are often similar in their effects. It is not necessarily a good result to save a marriage which is unsatisfactory to both partners, but the ill effects of divorce on the couple and their children should clearly be taken into account. Couple therapy can be usefully combined with individual therapy, either psychotherapeutic or with medication, and in some cases of psychosis couple therapy can make a significant reduction in relapse rate. Couple therapy cannot necessarily be expected to produce total and lasting removal of relationship problems or of individual symptoms, but in many couples after therapy there is a significant improvement in both. In many research studies this improvement has been shown to last for over a year, and if the couple can learn better ways of tackling new problems the relationship may become quite stable over a longer period of time.

Eating disorders

Management

Anorexia nervosa

Out-patient psychotherapy
Counselling or psychotherapy is effective if there has not been too much weight loss (namely less than 25 per cent). Specialist psychotherapy such as cognitive analytical therapy or modified dynamic therapy is more effective than supportive psychotherapy. Frequently the therapy has to be continued long term. It is important that this is supplemented by regular medical monitoring. It is helpful to have the family of patients under the age of 17 years involved in the treatment. Parental counselling is as effective and more acceptable to the family than family therapy.

In-patient treatment
This is necessary for those with severe weight loss. Staff with expertise in the management of eating disorders can provide a judicious mixture of psychotherapy and nutritional support. In extreme circumstances, people may be detained under the Mental Health Act.

Bulimia nervosa

The Royal College of Psychiatrist's Report recommends a stepped approach to treatment. Low-intensity interventions such as self-help manuals, groups, or guided self-care are useful in the first instance. Medium-term interventions such as cognitive behavioural or interpersonal therapy require more specialist skills. Patients with personality difficulties, for example the multi-impulsive or borderline patient, or those with additional physical morbidity such as diabetes mellitus may need long-term psychotherapy or in-patient treatment.

Investigations recommended for eating disorders on initial assessment

- full blood count (cells reduced: WBC > RBC > platelets)
- urea and electrolytes (low potassium, magnesium, calcium and phosphate; high bicarbonate)
- liver function test (all enzymes raised in severe starvation) and protein (decrease rare but sign poor prognosis)
- electrocardiogram (QT lengthening, μ wave)
- bone density (osteoporosis).

Treatment

Treatment must address the psychological aspects of anorexia and bulimia nervosa as well as the eating behaviour Refeeding alone may be successful in short-term weight restoration, but is usually ineffective in the long term.

Learning difficulties

Learning disability is not a disease: it does not respond to medical treatment. The appropriate treatment is that for the underlying mental condition (if any).

Drugs do not control primary behavioural disturbances: they may make behaviours much worse.

- Always carry out a physical examination. Refer for medical or surgical advice if pain is apparent. General diagnostic screening should be undertaken if there are signs of physical ill-health.

- Offer treatment appropriate to the underlying mental condition (if any). Sedation may be necessary to control the violently disturbed patient: caution is necessary in view of the frequent co-existence of epilepsy; Lorazepam is probably the safest sedative (2 mg orally, IV, or IM).

- Do **not** initiate regular neuroleptic medication.

Screening for specific syndromes of learning disability is generally pointless. Specialist investigations are best left to the specialist services. Long-term care in hospital is not an option.

11
Things you need to know about

Mental health act 1983 (MHA) (see table 11.01)

A working knowledge of the MHA is essential for all psychiatrists. This section summarizes some of the things you will need to know about most frequently. More details are to be found in the Code of Practice 1993.[1]

Section 1: definitions

Mental disorder is defined as: 'mental illness, arrested or incomplete development of mind, psychopathic disorder and any other disorder or disability of mind'.

Four categories of mental disorder are specified as follows:

1. **Mental illness** is not defined

2. **Severe mental impairment**: 'a state of arrested or incomplete development of mind which includes severe impairment of intelligence and social functioning and is associated with abnormally aggressive or seriously irresponsible conduct on the part of the person concerned'.

3. **Mental impairment**: is defined in the same way as severe mental impairment except that the phrase 'severe impairment' is replaced by 'significant impairment'.

4. **Psychopathic disorder**: 'a persistent disorder or disability of mind (whether or not including significant impairment of intelligence) which results in abnormally aggressive or seriously irresponsible conduct on the part of the person concerned.'

NB: Acute intoxication, substance dependence, or sexual preference disorders alone do not qualify for these criteria.

[1] Code of Practice. Mental Health Act 1983. HMSO, London: 1993.

Assessment prior to admission to hospital

As well as satisfying the criteria for mental disorder a patient may be compulsorily admitted under the MHA in the interests of his own health, **or** safety, **or** for the protection of others.

The code of practice also says that the following criteria should be considered:

- nature of illness/behaviour disorder
- patients wishes and views
- social and family circumstances
- views of patient, relatives and close friends about the likely course of the illness, the reliability of this, and any impact on them of a deterioration
- needs of family/cohabitees and the burden on them if not admitted under the Act
- need for protection of others — including past history, risk, and reliability of others to cope
- the appropriateness of guardianship
- impact of compulsory admission on patient's life after discharge
- the interests of the patients's own health and if there is any evidence that their mental health would deteriorate if no treatment received
- reliable evidence of risk to others and its nature and degree
- willingness and ability to cope with this risk by cohabitees.

If the patient is subject to the effects of sedative medication, or the short-term effects of drugs or alcohol, the *approved social worker* (ASW) should wait to apply for compulsory admission until the effects have abated, unless this is impossible because of the patient's disturbed behaviour. The ASW is responsible for co-ordinating the process of assessment and implementing the decision for application.

The **doctor** is responsible for:

- deciding if the patient is suffering from a mental disorder within the meaning of the Act, its seriousness, and the need for further assessment and/or treatment in hospital

- specifically addressing legal criteria for admission
- ensuring that a bed is available.

The doctors and ASWs, retain final responsibility, but should, wherever possible, consult colleagues; for example, CPNs.

Section 2 pointers

The following are indications for issuing a Section 2 notice:

- Where the diagnosis and prognosis of a patient's condition is unclear.
- There is a need to carry out an in-patient assessment in order to formulate a treatment plan.
- Where a judgement is needed as to whether the patient will accept treatment on a voluntary basis following admission.
- Where a judgement has to be made as to whether a particular treatment proposal, which can only be administered to the patient under Part IV of the Act, is likely to be effective.
- Where a patient who has already been assessed, and who has been previously admitted compulsorily under the Act, is judged to have changed since the previous admission and needs further assessment.
- Where the patient has not previously been admitted to hospital either compulsorily or informally.

Section 3 pointers

The following are indications for issuing a section 3 notice:

- Where a patient has been admitted in the past, is considered to need compulsory admission for the treatment of a mental disorder which is already known to his clinical team, and has been assessed in the recent past by that team.
- Where a patient already admitted under Section 2 and who is assessed as needing further medical treatment for mental disorder under the Act at the conclusion of his detention under

Section 2 is unwilling to remain in hospital informally and to consent to the medical treatment.

- Where a patient is detained under Section 2 and assessment points to a need for treatment under the Act for a period beyond the 28-day detention period allowed under Section 2. In such circumstances an application for detention under Section 3 should be made at the earliest opportunity and should not be delayed until the end of Section 2 detention. Changing a patient's detention status from Section 2 to Section 3 will not deprive him of a Mental Health Review Tribunal hearing if the change takes place after a valid application has been made to the Tribunal, but before it has been heard. The patient's rights to apply for a Tribunal under Section 66(1)(b) in the first period of detention after his change of status are unaffected.

Capacity and consent to treatment

Common law applies to all patients, detained or informal. Therefore, valid consent is required from a patient before medical treatment can be given, except where the law provides authority to treat him/her without consent.

It is the personal responsibility of any doctor proposing to treat a patient to determine whether the patient has the capacity to give a valid consent. In order to have capacity an individual must be able to understand:

- the nature of the proposed treatment
- why someone has said that he/she needs it
- the treatment's principal benefits and risks, and
- the consequences of not receiving the proposed treatment.

A person suffering from a mental disorder is not necessarily incapable of giving consent. The legal propositions regarding this are summarized in Lord Donaldson's judgment in *Re. T. (Adult: refusal of Medical Treatment)* (1992) All E.R. 649, 664 C.A. This presumes a capacity of an adult to refuse treatment if the reasons are 'rational or irrational, unknown or even non-existent'. An adult may be deprived of this capacity by long-term mental incapacity, retarded development, 'or by temporary factors such as unconsciousness or confusion or the effects of fatigue, shock, pain or drugs'. Doctors must consider the patient's capacity, taking into account the will of others vitiating the refusal, what treatment is being refused, and the circumstances in which it has arisen.

The junior doctor may be faced with the question of capacity in two common situations:

- a disturbed patient on a general ward refusing treatment
- a patient suffering from a mental disorder leading to behaviour that is an immediate serious danger to himself or to other people.

In the second case the MHA guidelines state that 'on rare occasions involving emergencies, where it is not possible immediately to apply the provisions of the MHA ... a patient ... may be given such treatment as represents the minimum necessary response to avert that danger'. In the first case, consideration should be given to the application of the MHA to the patient and both cases should ideally be discussed with seniors.

Consent to treatment (part IV of the Mental Health Act)

This applies to:

- Treatments prescribed for mental disorder,
- All formal patients except those who are detained under Sections 4, 5, 35, 135, and 136, subject to guardianship, or conditionally discharged: these patients have the right to refuse treatment as have informal patients, except in emergencies.

Part IV states that:

(i) any treatment can be given without the patient's consent unless the Mental Health Act or DHSS regulations specify otherwise

(ii) under section 57, psychosurgery and treatments specified in DHSS regulations as giving rise to special concern can only be given if

    (a) patient consents; and

    (b) a multidisciplinary panel appointed by the Mental Health Act Commission confirms that his consent is valid; and

(c) the doctor on the multidisciplinary panel certifies that the treatment should be given; before doing so he must consult two people, one a nurse and the other neither a nurse nor a doctor, who have been concerned with the patient's treatment.

Note: as the treatments specified in section 57 give rise to particular concern, this section applies to all formal and informal patients

(iii) under section 58, certain treatments can only be given if

(a) patient consents; or

(b) an independent doctor appointed by the Mental Health Act Commission confirms that treatment should be given; before doing so he must consult two people, one a nurse and the other neither a nurse nor a doctor, who have been concerned with the patient's treatment

Section 58 applies to treatments named in DHSS regulations (including electroconvulsive therapy, ECT). Medication can be given without the patient's consent for three months; after that it is subject to the safeguards laid down in Section 58.

Note under Section 62, any treatment for mental disorder can be given without consent in specific emergencies, subject to restrictions when a treatment is irreversible or hazardous.

Advocacy, rights and empowerment of patients using mental health services

Patients have a right to be treated with respect and the right to empathic staff. They also have the right to expect that the hospital ward will be a safe haven, where their legal and civil rights will be protected and upheld. The fact that a patient is on a Section of the Mental Health Act does not imply that the patient is not entitled to the exercise of his or her rights, but rather that in special circumstances that it would not be in the best interests of the patient and others for particular rights to be exercised.

A patient's mental health is likely to improve if he or she feels in control of their own life and able to take decisions either independently or in dialogue with a clinician. Patients often feel severely disempowered in mental health settings and a non-legal

Table 11.1

Section	Duration	Application	Procedures	Discharge
2 Admission for assessment	28 days maximum	ASW or nearest relative. Applicant must have seen patient within the previous 14 days	Two doctors must confirm that (a) patient is suffering from mental disorder of a nature or degree which warrants detention in hospital for assessment (or assessment followed by medical treatment) for at least a limited period; and (b) he ought to be detained in the interests of his own health or safety or with a view to the protection of others.	By any of the following: (a) RMO (b) hospital managers (c) nearest relative who must give 72 hours notice. RMO can prevent nearest relative discharging patient by making a report to the hospital managers (d) MHRT. Patient can apply to a tribunal within the first 14 days of detention.

Table 11.1 (Continued)

Section		Duration	Application	Procedures	Discharge
4	Admission for assessment in cases of emergency	72 hours maximum	ASW or nearest relative. Applicant must have seen patient within the previous 24 hours	One doctor must confirm that: (a) it is of 'urgent necessity' for the patient to be admitted and detained under Section 2; and (b) waiting for a second doctor to confirm the need for an admission under Section 2 would cause 'undesirable delay'.	
3	Admission for treatment	6 months, renewable for a further 6 months, then for one year at a time	By ASW or nearest relative. ASW must endeavour to identify the nearest relative, and take their wishes into account. However, the nearest relative cannot prevent an ASW from making an application (Section 26.1). [If nearest relative withholds	Two doctors must confirm that (a) patient is suffering from one of the four specified categories of mental disorder, a nature or degree which makes it appropriate for him to receive medical treatment in hospital; and (b) if patient is suffering from psychopathic disorder or mental impairment, such treatment is likely to 'alleviate or prevent a deterioration' of his condition; and	By any of the following: (a) RMO (b) hospital managers (c) nearest relative who must give 72 hours notice. RMO can prevent relative discharging patient by making a report to the hospital managers (d) MHRT. Patient can apply to a tribunal within

Table 11.1 (Continued)

Section	Duration	Application	Procedures	Discharge
		consent, ASW may apply to a County Court for the nearest relative's "displacement"].	(c) it is necessary for his own health or safety or for the protection of others that he receives such treatment and it cannot be provided unless he is detained under this section.	6 months of admission and during each subsequent renewal period.

Renewal: Under Section 20, RMO can renew a Section 3 detention order if original criteria still apply and treatment is likely to 'alleviate or prevent a deterioration' of patient's condition. In cases where patient is suffering from mental illness or severe mental impairment but treatment is not likely to alleviate or prevent a deterioration of his condition, detention may still be renewed if he is unlikely to be able to care for himself, to obtain the care he needs or to guard himself against serious exploitation.

Section	Duration	Application	Procedures	Discharge
5 (2)	72 hours maximum	Doctor of informal in-patient's treatment or nominated deputy (usually on-call Dr)	Reports to hospital managers that application for compulsory admission 'ought to be made'. Applies to inpatient's being treated for physical disorders but not those seen in Accident & Emergency. The nominated deputy should contact the rominated doctor or another consultant before using section 5 (2) where possible.	Should be converted to Section 2 or 3, or rescinded as soon as possible.

advocate (from the Community Health Council or Advocacy Organisation) can often help, in a non-adversarial way, to resolve conflicts and give the patient a stronger sense of control and personal autonomy.

Issues discussed at these meetings may include choice of medication, diagnosis, care plan, development and evaluation of the relationship with particular practitioners, criticism of the ward or mental health centre environment, and discussion about discharge and post-discharge arrangements. A patient may also wish to make a complaint. All patients are entitled to have an advocate with them at any time they choose, including during Management and Ward Rounds and case reviews.

Details of the patient's civil rights should be easily accessible on hospital wards and premises, reinforced regularly and always upheld. These rights include having access to the 'Patients Charter', national and local Mental Health Services Charters, and information about access to the Hospital Mental Health Managers, the Mental Health Act Commission, the Community Health Council, and local solicitors who specialize in mental health work.

Patients who are black or from an ethnic minority community and patients who have any type of disability have precisely the same rights as other patients and must not be denied services through poor communication or inaccessibility to services. Interpreters and advocates can assist to transform potentially difficult consultations into creative engagements, where the patient and doctor benefit from the clinical value of targeted advocacy.

The right of a patient to express his or her sexual orientation without fear of a pejorative or inappropriate response from medical staff should be seen as empowering and consistent with the responsibility of doctors to reinforce a patient's self-esteem and self-respect.

Patients involved in criminal proceedings (Part III)

Hospital order (Section 37)

Duration
Initially this lasts for six months, is then renewable for a further six months, then yearly.

Procedure

In the case of a convicted offender, a Hospital Order can be made by a Crown or Magistrates' court in place of a prison sentence. (Offences include manslaughter but not murder.) Magistrates' court need not record a conviction if satisfied that the offender was suffering from mental illness or severe mental impairment at the time of the offence.

A Hospital Order requires evidence from two doctors that:

- the offender is suffering from one of the specified categories of mental disorder of a nature and degree which makes detention for medical treatment appropriate, and

- if suffering from psychopathic disorder or mental impairment, such treatment is likely to 'alleviate or prevent a deterioration' of his/her condition, and

- taking into account all the relevant circumstances a hospital order is most appropriate.

Discharge

By the Responsible Medical Officer (RMO), hospital managers, or Medical Health Review Tribunal. (MHRT). One application is allowed between 6 and 12 months and then yearly. The case is automatically reconsidered by MHRT 3 years after the last tribunal referral.

Restriction Order (Section 41)

Duration

This may be specified by the court or be for a term without limit.

Procedure

A Restriction Order is made by a Crown court only after the imposition of a Hospital Order if

- this is necessary to protect the public from 'serious harm', and

- at least one of the doctors who made recommendations for the hospital order gave his/her evidence orally.

Discharge

Either the Home Secretary or the MHRT allow discharge (rules apply as for Section 37).

The Police and Criminal Evidence Act 1984

The Police and Criminal Evidence Act 1984 was designed to regulate police conduct and the admissibility of evidence in court. Sections 53–65 deal with the treatment and questioning of people in police custody.

If a detained person appears mentally disordered (defined according to Mental Health Act 1983 criteria), the police must ask an 'appropriate adult' to come to the police station. The concern is that a mentally disordered person will give evidence which is unreliable and/or self-incriminatory. Similar provision is made for juveniles. However, this does not apply in emergencies (for instance, where the risk to others can be reduced by questioning someone immediately).

The 'appropriate adult' may be a relative, carer, or someone who has worked with the mentally disordered, but it cannot be the person's solicitor. The adult cannot be employed by the police. The Code of Practice states that a well-informed professional may be preferable to an ill-informed relative, but also that the person's choice of adult is to be respected.

The 'appropriate adult' should be present during searches and questioning, observe fairness of interviews, advise the person being questioned, and facilitate communication. The person being questioned is entitled to consult privately with the appropriate adult at any time (this is often not respected).

The Act also makes provision that mentally disordered detainees should not be subject to voluntary searches (because of doubts about the quality of their consent). In all cases, the more stringent procedures which cover involuntary searches must be applied. If confessions made by mentally disordered people are used in evidence against them in court the judge must refer to the unreliability of such confessions in his or her summing up.

Emergency protection order (for children) (EPO)

Sometimes a psychiatric assessment of a child will reveal a dangerous and harmful situation so that emergency care is needed. If so, the duty social worker should be contacted urgently as well as the consultant in charge of the case.

The emergency protection order replaced the old Place of Safety Order under the Children and Young Person's Act 1969. It was felt, following the *Cleveland Inquiry*, that the place of safety order was used rather too indiscriminately, and that parental rights were too easily infringed.

An application for an Emergency Protection order can be made under Section 44 of the Children Act 1989. The court will make an order if there are reasonable grounds to believe that the child is likely to suffer significant harm, or cannot be seen in circumstances where he/she might be suffering significant harm. The court will wish to know why a child should be removed as a matter of urgency, and why parental cooperation should be dispensed with at this stage.

The duration is limited to 8 days, with a possible extension for a further 7 days. Applications to lift the order can be made between 72 hours and 8 days.

The person obtaining the order has limited parental responsibility. The court will decide about parental contact, and medical and psychiatric assessment.

The care programme approach

The Care Programme Approach (CPA) is an administrative measure which the Government instructed mental health and social services to introduce in 1991. It aims to guide good clinical practice, and to prevent patients from 'slipping through the net' of follow-up. The CPA is a central part of the Government's mental health policy.

It consists of four parts:

1. *Assessment of health and social care needs*: The systematic assessment of needs begins with a good psychiatric history,

which covers both the needs for diagnosis and treatment and needs for social care. Most patients with severe mental illnesses will have a wide range of needs (see pp. 236–7), and a full assessment will involve information obtained from informants: family, friends, professional and nonprofessional carers. Social workers, who have parallel assessment and 'care management' procedures, should be involved in more complex assessments, and these may be carried out jointly. A full needs assessment may require a multidisciplinary meeting. The risk of self-harm, self-neglect, or harm to others, should be assessed (see pp. 143–5; 134–41).

2. *A written care plan*: For in-patients, or out-patients who need multidisciplinary input, a care plan should be agreed at a ward round or CPA meeting with everyone who will be involved in implementing it. The plan should be agreed as far as possible with the patient, and with carers. For other patients, this might simply involve a plan for out-patient treatment being written in the notes after completing a history and examination, although even this should be discussed and agreed with the patient.

3. *Keyworker*: The keyworker has responsibility for the co-ordination of the care programme. If the patient moves to another area, a proper handover should be made by the keyworker to another team. The keyworker should be the professional with the closest relationship with the patient; this will often be a CPN or social worker, but could be the psychiatrist in training.

4. *Regular reviews*: The care plan should be usually be reviewed at least every 6 months, but the keyworker should be able to arrange for a review meeting with others involved in the patient's care if the care plan is not being effectively carried out. A register of names of patients needing reviews should be kept ('CPA register'), and reminders of the need for review issued.

Who should receive the CPA?

The CPA applies to all patients under the care of specialist psychiatric services. However, not every patient can or should have multidisciplinary team reviews. The CPA can be 'tiered', with most patients needing a 'minimal' CPA in which the basic elements of the CPA are represented by a written care plan in the notes, and where the out-patient doctor or CPA acts as keyworker and co-ordinates the follow-up. For other cases, an intermediate level of CPA can be applied, perhaps with brief reviews at team meetings or discussions between the staff involved; only more complex cases (including those on the supervision register see pp. 232–5) will require regular full multidisciplinary review meetings.

Communication and confidentiality

The care plan will often involve non-NHS bodies, for example voluntary sector housing, and good communication with them about the care plan is essential. However, the care plan is a medical record and the patient's right to confidentiality must be respected. Permission should be sought before communicating information outside the NHS; if this is not given, confidentiality can only be breached in exceptional circumstances, namely in the public interest, a decision which must be made by the consultant. The GP should always be informed.

Discharge from hospital

For in-patients, a CPA meeting should take place before discharge to ensure that the necessary community services will be in place. In the case of detained patients, this can also serve as a 'Section 117' meeting, where the aftercare required by Section 117 of the Mental Health Act is planned. If an adequate care plan cannot be put into practice, the patient should not be discharged.

Limitations of the CPA

The CPA requires considerable form filling and bureaucracy, which is only justifiable if it improves patient care. It can only help to target resources to those who need them most if resources are available, and if the CPA is properly 'tiered' rather than being applied equally to everyone.

Benefits

Assessing both medical and social needs fully, writing down plans of care, reviewing the plans, and ensuring that follow-up is provided are all basics of good medical practice. Done properly, the CPA encourages these.

The supervision register

The Supervision Register (SR) is an administrative measure which the Government instructed psychiatric services to introduce in 1994. It was felt to be necessary because of concerns, such as those expressed in the report of the *Inquiry into the Care of Christopher Clunis*, that the CPA was not being provided for those patients 'who may be at greatest risk and need most support'. It is part of the CPA, not a separate measure, and may be regarded as the most intensive tier of the CPA.

The Supervision Register is a list of names, held locally by the provider unit, of patients with a severe mental illness who are 'known to be at significant risk or potentially at significant risk of committing serious violence, or suicide or of serious self-neglect as the result of severe and enduring mental illness'. The register should be a subset of the CPA register, and should include the names of the patient, RMO, and keyworker as well as the nature of the risk, and details of the CPA (date of registration, components of the care plan, and review date).

Who should be on the supervision register?

Patients on the CPA should have a 'risk assessment' (see pp. 134–41) as part of their needs assessment (see pp. 236–7). The patient should be placed on the SR if it is judged that there is a significant risk of serious violence, self-harm, or self-neglect, and also that the risk occurs in circumstances which are possibly foreseeable in the particular case and can be addressed through a care plan (so although anyone who takes an overdose is at higher risk of subsequent self-harm, this would not in itself be a sufficient justification). Risk assessment is an inexact science, and the decision about what represents significant risk will be a matter of clinical judgement, usually in the context of a multidisciplinary team. Only a small proportion of patients (representing those at highest risk) on the team's case-load, should be on the SR if resources are to be targeted to them.

Discharge from hospital

If a care plan which addresses the risks the patient poses to themself or society cannot be put into practice, the patient should not be discharged. The risk assessment should help decision making about suitable accommodation and supports for the patient after discharge.

Confidentiality

The SR should identify those people where good communication will be of particular importance, and it is supposed to serve as a point of reference for health and social services staff to identify people at particular risk. However, it is a medical record and should be confidential. Usually it will be inappropriate or helpful to pass on the information that a patient is on the SR to anyone outside the psychiatric services. What should be communicated is information which will help others to manage the risk the patient poses, for example the indications of relapse, contexts in which the patient is more likely to be violent, and clear information on who to contact if the patient is causing concern. Patients should be told that they are on the SR, except in exceptional circumstances.

Limitations

Patients on the SR may have high needs for scarce resources (such as 24-hour residential care); if these resources are unavailable then targeting cannot help. Risk may not be sufficiently predictable for the SR to reduce the overall rates of violence and suicide significantly. Patients may be stigmatized as 'dangerous' on the basis of inaccurate predictions, and suffer stigma and difficulty in finding residential or other placements. Staff may not want to take on the responsibility of looking after patients on the SR, fearing they will be held responsible for subsequent episodes of violence.

Benefits

Although imprecise, risk assessment may be clinically worthwhile, and the SR may encourage people to assess and manage risk better. Resources may be targeted better to the most needy group of patients. If confidentiality is maintained, stigma can be avoided. Staff responsibility for patients' behaviour is not in fact increased by the existence of the SR, but by failure to assess and manage risk adequately.

Supervised discharge

Supervised discharge (SD) was introduced by the Mental Health (Patients in the Community) Act 1995, which amended the Mental Health Act 1983. It complements the Supervision Register, but is a statutory measure rather than an administrative one. It allows the RMO treating a patient under Sections 3, 37, 47, or 48 of the MHA to apply for powers of formal supervision of the patient after discharge from hospital, which will be exercised by a 'supervisor', typically a CPN acting as a keyworker.

Criteria for the application

The application is made by the RMO to the provider unit managers. The patient will already have satisfied the conditions for detention under the Sections given above: in addition, the RMO must believe that there will be a substantial risk of serious harm to the patient or to the safety of other people if the patient does not receive aftercare on discharge from hospital, and that the powers of supervised discharge are likely to help ensure that the patient receives aftercare. The aftercare will be delivered according to the CPA, and almost all patients who are subject to SD will be on the Supervision register (although not vice versa).

The application by the RMO must be supported by applications from another doctor approved under Section 12(2) — this could be the consultant providing community care (the 'Community RMO'), if different from the RMO, or the GP — and from an approved social worker. The application must include an agreed care plan.

The SD only takes effect once the patient is discharged both from hospital and from detention, so it does not apply while the patient is on leave of absence (Section 17). The patient has the right of appeal to a Mental Health Review Tribunal (but not to a managers' hearing). SD lasts for 6 months, and the RMO can apply to renew it for a further 6 months, then for 1 year at a time.

Responsibilities of the services

The RMO must consult the patient, the hospital team, the proposed supervisor (community keyworker), informal carers, the nearest relative, and social services about the application for SD. The care plan must be agreed with local social services, and should be agreed with others who will be involved in its implementation. The patient must be informed; he or she does not have to agree to be supervised, but in practice the care plan may be impossible to implement if the patient does not co-operate. The supervisor must monitor the provision of the care plan and the RMO must provide psychiatric treatment, and if the care plan is not working, they must consult the relevant parties and revise the plan.

Requirements of the patient

The patient can be required to reside in a particular place, to attend at set times for medical treatment, occupation, education, or training; the supervisor must be allowed access to the place of residence to see the patient.

Powers of the supervisor

The supervisor has the 'power to take and convey' the patient to home or to a place of treatment, with police or ambulance support if necessary. This can only be done if it is likely to result in the patient then co-operating with treatment, since the supervisor cannot prevent the patient from leaving the place of treatment as soon as he/she arrives, and the patient cannot be forced to take treatment. If necessary, the patient could be assessed for detention in hospital under Section 3.

Limitations

Although the procedure is elaborate, the powers are limited and cannot be used if they are ineffective, as they will be if the patient is determined not to co-operate with the care plan. They may restrict civil liberties without making it possible to deliver better care.

Benefits

There may be a small group of patients who are currently very difficult to care for who will respond to the more assertive treatment the supervisor can provide using SD.

Needs assessment

The assessment of need by both social and health services is a requirement of the Care Programme Approach. Social services are also required under the NHS and Community Care Act 1990 to provide an assessment of social care needs to all those who require one, including those with mental disorder — these types of assessment should overlap as much as is practicable.

Defining needs

Needs can be defined on a population or individual basis, and from the perspectives of politicians, clinicians, carers, and patients — clearly these will differ. A working definition of need, in the sense in which it is used in the CPA, is that a need exists where the patient 'is able in some way to benefit from care', where this care is medical or social. The needs are not limited to the care which happens to be available; a broader definition of need may suggest services which could be developed.

Need in severe mental illness

The needs for care of the severely mentally ill are often considerable, and involve physical, mental, and social needs. While a good psychiatric history and examination should identify many of these, some, particularly social care needs, may be insufficiently covered. A standardized instrument, the Camberwell Assessment of Needs (CAN[2]), identifies 22 areas of need to be explored in a full assessment (see Table 11.2). The instrument enables problems in these areas to be rated from interviews with the patient, or by the keyworker, in about 30 minutes, and distinguishes unmet needs from those already met by help from informal carers or statutory services.

Table 11.2   Camberwell Assessment of Needs

Accommodation	Alcohol
Food	Drugs
Household skills	Company of others
Self-care	Intimate relationships
Occupation	Sexual expression
Physical health	Child care
Psychotic symptoms	Basic education
Information about condition and treatment	Telephone
Psychological distress	Transport
Safety to self	Money
Safety to others	Welfare benefits

[2] Copies of the Camberwell Assessment of Needs are obtainable from PRiSM (Psychiatric Research in Service Measurement), Institute of Psychiatry, De Crespigny Park, Denmark Hill, London SE5 8AF. Tel. 0171–919–2610. Fax 0171–277–1462.

Community visits

This section discusses some practical aspects of patient contact by psychiatrists in non-medical settings. Community visiting is highly informative, enjoyable, and appreciated by both patients and carers. Visiting people at home provides an invaluable insight into the social context of the patient's psychopathology and their level of functioning. The techniques of assessment and management described in this book are equally applicable outside the hospital (for example in the patient's home, a hostel or day centre, a police station, or even the street). However, these settings are less predictable than the clinical or ward and more emotionally demanding. As a consequence some special considerations apply.

Patients may be seen in the community as part of the assessment process, for planned treatment or review, as an emergency intervention in a crisis, or in a formal Mental Health Act assessment. Family assessment and intervention may very usefully be carried out in the home. Care Programme Approach reviews are often held in non-medical settings. With the possible exception of the traditional consultant domiciliary consultation requested by the general practitioner, all home visiting should be part of the work of the multidisciplinary community mental health team. Home assessments by psychiatrists should generally be carried out together with colleagues in the team. Home treatment and review will be part of a previously agreed care plan. Emergency assessments should be carried out in accordance with locally agreed operational policies or protocols. 'Good practice' in the conduct of a Mental Health Act assessment is set out in a Code of Practice 1993,[3] with which, for medico-legal reasons, all psychiatrists is England and Wales should be familiar.

Planning the visit

The reasons for and expected outcome of any community visit should be identified. If hospital admission is the expected outcome

[3] Code of Practice. Mental Health Act 1983. HMSO, London 1993.

of an emergency assessment the availability of a bed should be confirmed before setting out. Alternatively, the possibilities of intensive community support to an acutely ill patient should be explored prior to the visit. If the patient is likely to require medication is a prescription available? A mobile telephone may be helpful if complex arrangements will have to be made. The visiting psychiatrist should have the maximum possible information. Prior to carrying out an emergency (or new patient) assessment informants should be contacted by telephone. Any documentation should be sought and read. It is helpful to know the exact nature of the community concerns before any doorstep assessment:

- What is the alleged psychopathology?
- What abnormal behaviours have others reported?
- What are the patient's documented risks to self or others?

The patient should generally be given notice of the visit, which should preferably take place at a mutually agreed time. The reason for and conduct of any unannounced visit should be very clearly thought out in advance. The journey to a visit should be planned: find out exactly where to go, how long it will take, and where to park. At night take a torch. If a colleague, carer, or the police are to attend the visit a rendezvous should be agreed. Arrangements for access to the home should be identified before the visit: if access is impossible consideration should be given to the use of Section 135 of the Mental Health Act. This requires the involvement of an ASW colleague.

Safety

The possible risks of any community visit should always be considered:

- Is the patient (and family) known to services?
- Is there any past history of violence or aggression?
- Is there a large dog in the house?

If there are any concerns about safety the psychiatrist should visit with a colleague from the team, the GP, or a person previously known to the patient. Unobtrusive police presence may be advisable during a Mental Health Act assessment. As a general principle, *another team member should know about any community visit*: community staff have been held hostage! If during a visit staff feel unsafe they should not hesitate to retreat. If, following a strategic retreat, there are concerns about the safety of other household members some plan of action should be drawn up, for example a follow-up telephone call or contact with the police.

Carrying out a visit

Any home visit should be carried out in a calm and confident manner. The psychiatrist is often expected to take the lead in the conduct of the visit, and should, therefore, be clear about the point of the visit. Communications should be clear and unambiguous. Certain courtesies should be observed, for example seeking permission to enter the house and establishing with the patient and any carer the purpose of the interview, its likely duration, and where it should be carried out. Introductions should be made. The composition of the household should be established: visitors should be sensitive to the needs of children in the home. When there are carers present they should be allowed to contribute to the discussion of the patient's problems, although rights to confidentiality should always be considered. It may be appropriate to interview the patient and carers separately. It is quite reasonable to ask the patient to turn off their television or remove their pet from the interview setting. If one aim of the visit is to assess the patient's level of functioning and home environment this should be carried out sensitively, although it is usually appropriate to share any concerns about their welfare with the patient. At the end of the visit a plan of further care should be negotiated with the patient and carer. Preferably the timing of any further home visit or outpatient contact should be agreed. Details of a contact person, address, and telephone number should be offered to the patient and carer. The referrer should be formally contacted following an assessment, which should be recorded in the case notes. It will often be helpful to carry out a short debriefing session with any accompanying colleague immediately after the visit, both to clarify the outcome of the visit and for emotional support.

Emergency and Mental Health Act assessments

The conduct of emergency assessments will reflect the treatment paradigms, resource base, and policies of the local service. There may be a Crisis Intervention Team capable of responding to requests from GPs, patients and carers, and community agencies for the assessment and treatment of people in psychosocial crisis. A service may be able to provide 24-hour home care for acutely psychotic patients as an alternative to in-patient admission, or may only be able to offer institution of treatment, intermittent home visits, and out-patient attendance. The general principles are set out above: careful planning (it is the more acute the situation, the more important it is), consideration of personal safety, calm conduct throughout the intervention, and appropriate follow-up. Access arrangements are crucial to effective emergency interventions.

Assessments for admission under the Mental Health Act should generally follow the 'good practice' guidelines set out in the Code of Practice, or its equivalent in other jurisdictions. The Code of Practice not only amplifies the criteria for compulsory admission set out in the Mental Health Act, but provides detail about the appropriate conduct of the assessment. Mental Health Act assessments are often unnecessarily chaotic and distressing for patient, carers, and the staff involved. Although a rapid response to a perceived crisis is often demanded, careful planning is always appropriate. The ASW has 'overall responsibility for co-ordinating the process of assessment and, where he decides to make an application, for implementing the decision' (Code of Practice 2.10). The psychiatrist (always approved under Section 12 of the Mental Health Act) may wish to review these plans before the assessment and should usually have made arrangements for the patient's admission to an appropriately staffed ward in the anticipation of a decision to admit either under the Mental Health Act or informally. An ambulance and, if necessary, the police should be in attendance. Assessment should be carried out jointly by the recommending doctors (the psychiatrist and usually the GP) and the ASW 'unless good reasons prevent it' (Code of Practice 2.2). The role of the ASW is spelt out in detail (2.11–2.17). The medical examination requires 'direct personal examination of the patient's mental state' and 'consideration of all available relevant medical information' (2.20). Examining doctors 'should always discuss the patient with each other' (2.21).

Although the majority of compulsory admissions 'require prompt action to be taken' the ASW has up to 14 days from first seeing the patient to making an application (2.26). Any decision not to make an application should be accompanied by plans to implement appropriate alternative arrangements. The ASW also has a duty to inform the nearest relative of the reasons for not making an application and their right to apply (2.27).

Home visits with elderly patients

If the patient is being assessed at home some inspection of the home circumstances should be made. This is an important part in evaluating the degree of risk posed to the patient (and possibly others). Remember that self-neglect is not diagnostic of any particular disorder and can occur in severe functional illness as well as dementia.

- Is the dwelling in a good state of repair and decoration?
- Is it secure?
- Are gas, electricity, and water supplies connected?
- Is there adequate heating and lighting?
- Is the gas ever left on unlit?
- If the patient smokes, is there evidence of the careless use of lighted cigarettes?
- Is the patient able to call for help if necessary (for example, by means of a centralized alarm system)?
- Is there enough food in the home to make, at least, small snacks/hot drinks?
- Is there evidence of urinary or faecal incontinence?
- Are any pets well cared for?

Appendix 1

Mini-Mental State Examination

(Folstein *et al.* (1975) *Journal of Psychiatric Research*, **12**, 189)

			Score	Points
Orientation				
1. What is the	Year?		...	1
	Season?		...	1
	Date?		...	1
	Day?		...	1
	Month?		...	1
2. Where are we?	Country?		...	1
	County?		...	1
	Town?		...	1
	Hospital?		...	1
	Floor?		...	1

Registration

3. Name three objects, one per second (e.g. BALL, FLAG, TREE).
   Then ask the patient all three after you have said them. Give one point for each correct answer.
   Repeat the words until patient learns all three ... 3

Attention and Concentration

4. Spell 'world' backwards: D L R O W ... 5

Recall

5. Ask for names of three objects learned in Q.3.
   Give one point for each correct answer. ... 3

Language

6. Point to a pencil and a watch.
   Ask the patient to name them as you point. ... 2

7. Ask the patient to repeat 'No ifs, ands or buts' ... 1

8. Ask the patient to read and obey the following:
   CLOSE YOUR EYES ... 1

Language

9. Ask the patient to carry out a three-stage
    command:
    'Take the paper in your right hand, fold it
    in half and put it on the floor.'   ...   3

10. Ask the patient to write a sentence of their own.
    (The sentence should contain a subject and
    an object and should make sense. Ignore
    spelling errors in scoring).   ...   1

11. Ask the patient to copy a design (2 overlapping
    pentagons. Give one point if all sides and
    angles are preserved and the intersecting
    sides form a quadrangle).   ...   1
                                                                  ___
                                          TOTAL   30

Appendix 2

Table A2.1 Antipsychotic drugs

Drug	Chemical group	Dose range (daily dose) Single daily dose unless stated (*)	Alternative licensed indications	Adverse effects (See data sheet for full details/ Appendix 4 for comparison)	Interactions	Cost
Chlorpromazine	Phenothiazine (Gp I — aliphatic)	25–1000 mg	Anxiety, nausea, agitation, hiccup, induction of hypothermia, violence, autism	Extrapyramidal effects, anticholinergic, sedation, hypotension, hypothermia, endocrine disorders, convulsions, jaundice, ECG change, blood dyscrasias	Sedatives, lithium, anticholinergics, anti-epileptics, sulphonylureas, cimetidine, antidepressants, dopamine (ant)agonists	£ 0.04/100 mg tablet

Table A2.1 (*Continued*)

Drug	Chemical group	Dose range (daily dose) Single daily dose indications unless stated (*)	Alternative licensed indications	Adverse effects (See data sheet for full details/ Appendix 4 for comparison)	Interactions	Cost
Promazine	Phenothiazine (Gp I — aliphatic)	400–800 mg	Agitation and restlessness in elderly NB Weak antipsychotic	As chlorpromazine	As chlorpromazine	£ 0.18/200 mg syrup
Thioridazine	Phenothiazine (Gp II — piperidine)	150–800 mg	Agitation, anxiety, violence, impulsive behaviour. Agitation and restlessness in the elderly	As chlorpromazine + pigmented retinopathy, ejaculatory dysfunction	As chlorpromazine	£ 0.06/100 mg tablet
Fluphenazine	Phenothiazine (Gp III — piperazine)	1–20 mg	Agitation, anxiety, violence	As chlorpromazine + depression reported	As chlorpromazine	£ 0.07/2.5 mg tablet

Drug	Class	Dose	Indications			Cost
Perphenazine	Phenothiazine (gp III — piperazine)	12–24 mg	Agitation, severe anxiety, violence	As chlorpromazine	As chlorpromazine	£ 0.20/4 mg tablet
Trifluoperazine	Phenothiazine (Gp III — piperazine)	10–50 mg (est) (maximum dose not stated by manufacturers)	Agitation, severe anxiety, violence	As chlorpromazine	As chlorpromazine	£ 0.04/5 mg tablet
Flupenthixol	Thioxanthine	6–18 mg	Depressive illness (low dose)	As chlorpromazine	As chlorpromazine	£ 0.14/3 mg tablet
Zuclopenthixol	Thioxanthine	20–150 mg	None	As chlorpromazine	As chlorpromazine	£ 0.08/10 mg tablet
Haloperidol	Butyrophenone	1.5–120 mg	Agitation, severe anxiety, violence, tics, nausea, hiccup, mania, Gilles de Tourette	As chlorpromazine	As chlorpromazine + fluoxetine, astemizole, terfenadine	£ 0.08/5 mg tablet

Table A2.1 (Continued)

Drug	Chemical group	Dose range (daily dose) Single daily dose unless stated (*)	Alternative licensed indications	Adverse effects (See data sheet for full details/ Appendix 4 for comparison)	Interactions	Cost
Droperidol	Butyrophenone	20–120 mg* (4 times per day) (sedative)	Anaesthesia, mania, nausea. NB For *acute* treatment only	As chlorpromazine + depression	As chlorpromazine	£ 0.25/10 mg tablet
Benperidol	Butyrophenone	0.25–1.5 mg* (2 times per day)	Deviant social/ sexual behaviour NB Not licensed for schizophrenia/ psychoses	As chlorpromazine	As chlorpromazine	£ 0.26/0.25 mg tablet
Sulpiride	Substituted benzamide	400–2400 mg* (2 times per day)	None	As chlorpromazine, jaundice and skin reactions less common	As chlorpromazine	£ 0.20/200 mg tablet
Pimozide	Diphenylbutyl piperidine	2–20 mg	Mania, hypochondriacal	As chlorpromazine + serious cardiac	As chlorpromazine	£ 0.16/2 mg tablet

		psychosis		arrhythmias (monitor plasma potassium), depression	+ diuretics, any cardioactive drug — this includes other antipsychotics and tricyclics	
Loxapine	Dibenzoxazepine	20–250 mg* (2 times per day)	None	As chlorpromazine + nausea, dyspnoea, ptosis, polydipsia, paraesthesia. Few endocrine effects reported	As chlorpromazine	£ 0.10/10 mg capsule
Risperidone	Benzisoxazole	2–16 mg* (2 times per day)	None	As chlorpromazine + agitation, abdominal pain, fatigue, anxiety, nausea, rhinitis	As chlorpromazine	£ 1.95/3 mg tablet
Sertindole (Consultant only)	Imidazolidinone	12–24 mg/day See Product Data Sheet for full details	None	As chlorpromazine + nasal congestion, reduced ejaculatory volume	As chlorpromazine + all drugs which inhibit CYP2D6, e.g. fluoxetine, paroxetine	£3.66/12 mg tablet

Table A2.1 *(Continued)*

Drug	Chemical group	Dose range (daily dose) Single daily dose unless stated (*)	Alternative licensed indications	Adverse effects (See data sheet for full details/ Appendix 4 for comparison)	Interactions	Cost
Clozapine	Dibenzodiazepine	25–900 mg* (2 times per day)	None	As chlorpromazine + hypersalivation, delirium, incontinence, myocarditis, neutropenia, fatal agranulocytosis (see Appendix 4)	As chlorpromazine + all drugs which depress leucopoiesis: e.g. cytotoxic agents, sulphonamides, chloramphenicol, carbamazepine, phenothiazines. Fluoxetine and risperidone increase clozapine plasma levels	£ 1.79/100 mg tablet

Table A2.2 Antipsychotic drugs: relative adverse effects

Drug	Sedation	Extra-Pyramidal	Anti-Cholinergic	Hypotension	Cardiac toxicity
Chlorpromazine	+++	++	++	+++	++
Promazine	+++	+	++	++	+
Thioridazine	+++	+	+++	+++	++
Fluphenazine	+	+++	++	+	+
Perphenazine	+	+++	+	+	+
Trifluoperazine	+	+++	–	+	+
Flupenthixol	+	++	++	+	+
Zuclopenthixol	++	++	++	+	+
Haloperidol	+	+++	+	+	+
Droperidol	++	+++	+	+	+

Table A2.2 *(Continued)*

Drug	Sedation	Extra-Pyramidal	Anti-Cholinergic	Hypotension	Cardiac toxicity
Benperidol	+	++	+	+	+
Sulpiride	–	+	+/–	–	–
Pimozide	+	+	+	+++	+++
Loxapine	++	++	+	++	+
Clozapine	+++	–	+++	+++	+
Risperidone*	+	–	+	++	–

+++, high incidence/severity;++, moderate;+, low;–, very low/none.
* akathisia common with risperidone.

Appendix 3

Table A3.1 Antipsychotic Depot Injections (Suggested doses and frequencies)

Drug	Trade name	Test dose (mg)	Dose range (mg/ week)	Dosing interval (weeks)	Comments
Flupenthixol decanoate	Depixol	20	12.5– 400	2–4	Mood elevating; may worsen agitation
Fluphenazine decanoate	Modecate	12.5	6.25– 50	2–5	Avoid in depression. High EPSE[a]
Haloperidol decanoate	Haldol	25*	12.5– 75	4	High EPSE[a], low incidence of sedation
Pipothiazine palmitate	Piportil	25	12.5– 50	4	Lower incidence of EPSE[a]
Zuclopenthixol decanoate	Clopixol	100	100– 600	2–4	Useful in agitation and aggression

Notes

- Give 25 or 50 per cent stated doses in the elderly.

- After the test dose, wait 4–10 days before starting titration to maintenance therapy.

- Dose range is given in mg/week for convenience only — avoid using shorter dose intervals than those recommended except in exceptional circumstances, e.g. long interval necessitates high volume (> 3–4 ml) injection.

- EPSE, extrapyramidal side-effects.

* Test dose not stated by manufacturer.

Appendix 4

Table A4.1   Clozapine: management of adverse effects

Adverse effect	Timecourse	Action
Sedation	First 4 weeks. May persist, but usually wears off.	Give smaller dose in the mornings. Some patients can only cope with single nighttime dosing. Reduce dose if necessary.
Hypersalivation	First 4 weeks. May persist, but usually wears off. Often very troublesome at night.	Give hyoscine 300 μg (Kwells®) chewed and swallowed at night. Propantheline 15 mg three times per day may be used but worsens anticholinergic effects. Pirenzepine may be tried. Patients do not always mind excess salivation: treatment not always required.
Constipation	Usually persists	Recommend high fibre diet. Bulk-forming laxatives +/– stimulants may be used.
Hypotension	First 4 weeks	Advise patient to take time when standing up. Reduce dose or slow down rate of increase. If severe, consider moclobemide and Bovril.
Tachycardia	First 4 weeks, but often persists.	Often occurs if dose escalation is too rapid. Inform patient that it is not dangerous. Give small dose of beta-blocker if necessary.
Weight gain	Usually during the first year of treatment.	Dietary counselling is essential. Advice may be more effective if given before weight gain occurs. Weight gain is common and often profound (> 2 stone, 12.7 kg).

Table A4.1 (Continued)

Adverse effect	Timecourse	Action
Fever	First 3 weeks	Give antipyretic. NB. This fever is not usually related to blood dyscrasias.
Seizures	May occur at any time.	Dose related. Consider prophylactic valproate* if on high dose. After a seizure — withhold clozapine for one day. Restart at reduced dose. Give sodium valproate
Nausea	First 6 weeks	May give antiemetic. Avoid prochlorperazine and metoclopramide (EPSE).
Neutropenia/ agranulocytosis	First 18 weeks (but may occur at any time).	Stop clozapine; admit to hospital.

* Usual dose is 1000–2000 mg/day. Plasma levels may be useful as a rough guide to dosing — aim for 50–100 mg/L. Use of modified release preparation [sodium valproate (as valproate and valproic acid: Epilim Chrono)] may aid compliance: can be given once daily and may be better tolerated.

Appendix 5

Table A5.1 Equivalent doses of neuroleptics

Drug	Equivalent dose (consensus) (mg/day)	Range of values in literature (mg/day)
Chlorpromazine	100	—
Thioridazine	100	75–100
Fluphenazine	2	2–5
Trifluoperazine	5	2.5–5
Flupenthixol	3	2–3
Zuclopenthixol	25	25–60
Haloperidol	3	1.5–5
Droperidol	4	1–4
Sulpiride	200	200–270
Pimozide	2	2
Loxapine	10	10–25
Clozapine	50	50–90
Risperidone	2	?
Fluphenazine depot	5/week	1–12.5/week
Pipothiazine depot	10/week	10–12.5/week
Flupenthixol depot	10/week	10–20/week
Zuclopenthixol depot	100/week	40–100/week
Haloperidol depot	15/week	5–25/week

Note: All values should be regarded as approximate.

Table A5.2   Oral/parenteral dose equivalents

Drug	Oral dose (mg)	Equivalent IM or IV dose (mg)
Benzodiazepines		
Diazepam	10	10
Lorazepam	4	4
Antipsychotics		
Chlorpromazine	100	25–50
Droperidol	10	7.5
Haloperidol	10	5
Promazine	200	200
Anticholinergics		
Procyclidine	10	7.5

Note: Because of the variation in bioavailability with some drugs, prescriptions should always specify the dose *and* a single route of administration; for example, Droperidol 10 mg IM Q6H PRN

Table A5.3   Maximum daily doses — antipsychotics

Drug	Maximum dose (mg/day)
Chlorpromazine	1000
Thioridazine	800 (see BNF)
Fluphenazine	20
Trifluoperazine	None
Flupenthixol	18
Zuclopenthixol	150
Haloperidol	120
Droperidol	120
Sulpiride	2400
Pimozide	20
Loxapine	250
Clozapine	900
Risperidone	16
Fluphenazine depot	50/week
Pipothiazine depot	50/week
Haloperidol depot	300 every 4 weeks
Flupenthixol depot	400/week
Zuclopenthixol depot	600/week

Note: Doses above these maxima should only be used in extreme circumstances: there is no evidence for improved efficacy. Always follow RCP guidelines.

Appendix 6

The AUDIT questionnaire (screen for alcohol problems)

Circle the number that comes closest to the patient's answer.

1. **How often do you have a drink containing alcohol?**
   - (0) Never
   - (1) Monthly or less
   - (2) Two to four times a month
   - (3) Two to three times a week
   - (4) Four or more times a week

2.* **How many drinks containing alcohol do you have on a typical day when you are drinking? (Code Number of Standard Drinks)**
   - (0) 1 or 2
   - (1) 3 or 4
   - (2) 5 or 6
   - (3) 7 or 8
   - (4) 10 or more

3. **How often do you have six or more drinks on one occasion?**
   - (0) Never
   - (1) Less than monthly
   - (2) Monthly
   - (3) Weekly
   - (4) Daily or almost daily

4. **How often during the last year have you found that you were not able to stop drinking once you had started?**
   - (0) Never
   - (1) Less than monthly
   - (2) Monthly
   - (3) Weekly
   - (4) Daily or almost daily

5. **How often during the last year have you failed to do what was normally expected from you because of drinking?**
   - (0) Never
   - (1) Less than monthly
   - (2) Monthly
   - (3) Weekly
   - (4) Daily or almost daily

259

The AUDIT questionnaire (screen for alcohol problems) (Continued)

6. **How often during the last year have you needed a first drink in the morning to get yourself going after a heavy drinking session?**

| (0) Never | (1) Less than monthly | (2) Monthly | (3) Weekly | (4) Daily or almost daily |

7. **How often during the last year have you had a feeling of guilt or remorse after drinking?**

| (0) Never | (1) Less than monthly | (2) Monthly | (3) Weekly | (4) Daily or almost daily |

8. **How often during the last year have you been unable to remember what happened the night before because you had been drinking?**

| (0) Never | (1) Less than monthly | (2) Monthly | (3) Weekly | (4) Daily or almost daily |

9. **Have you or someone else been injured as a result of your drinking?**

| (0) No | (1) Yes, but not in the last year | | (4) Yes, during the last year |

10. **Has a relative or friend or a doctor or other health worker, been concerned about your drinking or suggested you cut down?**

| (0) No | (1) Yes, but not in the last year | | (4) Yes, during the last year |

* In determining the response categories it has been assumed that one 'drink' contains 10 g alcohol. In countries where the alcohol content of a standard drink differs by more than 25% from 10 g, the response category should be modified accordingly.

Appendix 7
World Health Organization (1992): The ICD-10 Classification of Mental and Behavioural Disorders: Clinical Descriptions and Diagnostic Guidelines. World Health Organization: Geneva

When trying to understand the overall structure of the classification, or how disorders are related to each other, it is helpful to be able to see the whole classification at a glance, and also to see it arranged in different degrees of detail. This chart (both sides) shows the whole classification, going down to the 5th character whenever it occurs. On the last part of the reverse side of the chart, the classification is shown in its simplest form by means of the headings of the ten blocks, F00–F99, and also at the intermediate 3-character level.

LIST OF CATEGORIES

(Categories present only in the DCR-10 are marked with a star*)

F00–F09
Organic, including symptomatic, mental disorders

F00   Dementia in Alzheimer's disease
F00.0 Dementia in Alzheimer's disease with early onset
F00.1 Dementia in Alzheimer's disease with late onset
F00.2 Dementia in Alzheimer's disease, atypical or mixed type

F00.8 Dementia in Alzheimer's disease, unspecified

F01   Vascular Dementia
F01.0 Vascular dementia of acute onset
F01.1 Multi-infarct dementia
F01.2 Subcortical vascular dementia
F01.3 Mixed cortical and subcortical vascular dementia
F01.8 Other vascular dementia
F01.9 Vascular dementia, unspecified

F02   Dementia in other diseases classified elsewhere
F02.0 Dementia in Pick's disease
F02.1 Dementia in Creutzfeld–Jakob disease
F02.2 Dementia in Huntington's disease
F02.3 Dementia in Parkinson's disease
F02.4 Dementia in human immunodeficiency virus (HIV) disease
F02.8 Dementia in other specified diseases classified elsewhere

F03   Unspecified dementia
A fifth character may be used to specify dementia in F00–F03, as follows:

.x0 Without additional symptoms

.x1 With other symptoms, predominantly delusional

.x2 With other symptoms, predominantly hallucinatory

.x3 With other symptoms, predominantly depressive

.x4 With other mixed symptoms

* A sixth character may be used to indicate the severity of the dementia:
*.xx0 Mild
*.xx1 Moderate
*.xx2 Severe

F04   Organic amnesic syndrome, not induced by alcohol and other psychoactive substances

F05   Delirium, not induced by alcohol and other psychoactive substances

F05.0   Delirium, not superimposed on dementia, so described

F05.1   Delirium, superimposed on dementia, so described

F05.8   Other delirium

F05.9   Delirium, unspecified

F06   Other mental disorders due to brain damage and dysfunction and to physical disease

F06.0   Organic hallucinosis

F06.1   Organic catatonic disorder

F06.2   Organic delusional (schizophrenia-like) disorder

F06.3   Organic mood (affective) disorder

.30   Organic manic disorder

.31   Organic bipolar disorder

.32   Organic depressive disorder

.33   Organic mixed affective disorder

F06.4   Organic anxiety disorder

F06.5   Organic dissociative disorder

F06.6   Organic emotionally labile (asthenic) disorder

F06.7   Mild cognitive disorder

.70   Not associated with a physical disorder

.71   Associated with a physical disorder

F06.8   Other specified mental disorders due to brain damage and dysfunction and to physical disease

F06.9   Unspecified mental disorders due to brain damage and dysfunction and to physical disease

F07   Personality and behavioural disorders due to brain disease, damage and dysfunction

F07.0   Organic personality disorder

F07.1   Postencephalitic syndrome

F07.2   Postconcussional syndrome

F07.8   Other organic personality and behavioural disorders due to brain disease, damage and dysfunction

F07.9   Unspecified mental disorders due to brain disease, damage and dysfunction

F09   Unspecified organic or symptomatic mental disorder

**F10–F19
Mental and behavioural disorders due to psychoactive substance use**

F10.–   Mental and behavioural disorders due to use of alcohol

F11.–   Mental and behavioural disorders due to use of alcohol

F12.–	**Mental and behavioural disorders due to use of cannabinoids**		.05	With coma
			.06	With convulsions
F13.–	**Mental and behavioural disorders due to use of sedatives or hypnotics**		.07	Pathological intoxication

F1x.1 Harmful use

F1x.2 Dependence syndrome

F14.– **Mental and behavioural disorders due to use of cocaine**

    .20 Currently abstinent

       200 Early remission

F15.– **Mental and behavioural disorders due to use of other stimulants, including caffeine**

       201 Partial remission

       202 Full remission

F16.– **Mental and behavioural disorders due to use of hallucinogens**

    .21 Currently abstinent, but in a protected environment

F17.– **Mental and behavioural disorders due to use of tobacco**

    .22 Currently on a clinically supervised maintenance or replacement regime (controlled dependence)

F18.– **Mental and behavioural disorders due to use of volatile solvents**

    .23 Currently abstinent, but receiving treatment with aversive or blocking drugs

F19.– **Mental and behavioural disorders due to multiple drug use and use of other psychoactive substances**

    .24 Currently using the substance (active dependence)

       .240 Without physical features

Four-, Five- and six-character categories are used to specify the clinical conditions as follows, and diagnostic criteria particular to each psychoactive substance are provided where appropriate for acute intoxication and withdrawal state:

       .241 With physical features

    .25 Continuous use

    .26 Episodic use (dipsomania)

F1x.3 Withdrawal state

    .30 Uncomplicated

    .31 With convulsions

F1x.0 Acute intoxication

    .00 Uncomplicated

    .01 With trauma or other bodily injury

    .02 With other medical complications

    .03 With delirium

    .04 With perceptual distortions

F1x.4 Withdrawl state with delirium
  .40 Without convulsions
  .41 With convulsions
F1x5 Psychotic disorder
  .50 Schizophrenia-like
  .51 Predominantly delusional
  .52 Predominantly hallucinatory
  .53 Predominantly polymorphic
  .54 Predominantly depressive psychotic
  .55 Predominantly manic psychotic symptoms
  .56 Mixed
F1x.6 Amnesic syndrome
F1x.7 Psychotic disorder
  .70 Flashbacks
  .71 Personality or behavioural disorder
  .72 Residual affective disorder
  .73 Dementia
  .74 Other persisting cognitive disorder
  .75 Late-onset psychotic disorder
F1x.8 Other mental and behavioural disorders
F1x.9 Unspecified mental and behavioural disorder

F20-F29
Schizophrenia, schizotypal and delusional disorders

F20 Schizophrenia
F20.0 Paranoid schizophrenia
F20.1 Hebephrenic schizophrenia
F20.2 Catatonic schizophrenia
F20.3 Undifferentiated schizophrenia
F20.4 Post-schizophrenic depression
F20.5 Residual schizophrenia
F20.6 Simple schizophrenia
F20.8 Other schizophrenia
F20.9 Schizophrenia, unspecified

A fifth character may be used to classify course:
  .x0 Continuous
  .x1 Episodic with progressive deficit
  .x2 Episodic with stable deficit
  .x3 Episodic remittent
  .x4 Incomplete remission
  .x5 Complete remission
  .x8 Other
  .x9 Course uncertain, period of observation too short

F21 Schizotypal disorder

F22 Persistant delusional disorders
F22.0 Delusional disorders
F22.8 Other persistent delusional disorders
F22.9 Persistent delusional disorder, unspecified

F23 Acute and transient psychotic disorders
F23.0 Acute polymorphic psychotic disorder without symptoms or schizophrenia
F23.1 Acute polymorphic psychotic disorder with symptoms of schizophrenia
F23.2 Acute schizophrenia-like psychotic disorder
F23.3 Other acute predominantly delusional psychotic disorder
F23.8 Other acute and transient psychotic disorder
F23.9 Acute and transient psychotic disorder, unspecified

A fifth character may be used to classify course:

.x0 Without associated acute stress

.x1 With associated acute stress

F24 Induced delusional disorder

F25 Schizoaffective disorders
F25.0 Schizoaffective disorder, manic type
F25.1 Schizoaffective disorder, depressive type
F25.2 Schizoaffective disorder, mixed type
F23.8 Other schizoaffective disorders
F23.9 Schizoaffective disorder, unspecified

* A fifth character may be used to classify the following subtypes:

*.x0 Concurrent affective and schizophrenic symptoms only

*.x1 Concurrent affective and schizophrenic symptoms plus persistence of the schizophrenic symptoms beyond the duration of the affective symptoms

F28 Other non-organic psychotic disorders

F29 Unspecified non-organic psychosis

F30–F39
Mood [affective] disorders

F30 Manic episode
F30.0 Hypomania
F30.1 Mania without psychotic symptoms
F30.2 Mania with psychotic symptoms

*.20 With mood-congruent psychotic symptoms

*.21 With mood-incongruent psychotic symptoms
F30.8 Other manic episodes
F30.9 Manic episode, unspecified

F31 Bipolar affective disorder
F31.0 Bipolar affective disorder, current episode hypomanic
F31.1 Bipolar affective disorder, current episode manic without psychotic symptoms
F31.2 Bipolar affective disorder, current episode manic with psychotic symptoms

*.20 With mood congruent psychotic symptoms

*.21 With mood-incongruent psychotic symptoms
F31.3 Bipolar affective disorder, current episode mild or moderate depression

.30 Without somatic syndrome

.31 With somatic syndrome
F31.4 Bipolar affective disorder, current episode severe depression without psychotic symptoms
F31.5 Bipolar affective disorder, current episode severe depression with psychotic symptoms

*.50 With mood-congruent psychotic symptoms

*.51 With mood-incongruent psychotic symptoms
F31.6 Bipolar affective disorder, current episode mixed
F31.7 Bipolar affective disorder, currently in remission
F31.8 Other bipolar affective disorders
F31.9 Bipolar affective disorder, unspecified

F32 Depressive episode
F32.0 Mild depressive episode

	.00	Without somatic syndrome
	.01	With somatic syndrome
F32.1		Moderate depressive episode
	.10	Without somatic syndrome
	.11	With somatic syndrome
F32.2		Severe depressive episode without psychotic symptoms
F32.3		Severe depressive episode with psychotic symptoms
	*.30	With mood-congruent psychotic symptoms
	*.31	With mood-incongruent psychotic symptoms
F32.8		Other depressive episodes
F32.9		Depressive episode, unspecified

F33 Recurrent depressive disorder

F33.0		Recurrent depressive disorder, current episode mild
	.00	Without somatic syndrome
	.01	With somatic syndrome
F33.1		Recurrent depressive disorder, current episode moderate
	.10	Without somatic syndrome
	.11	With somatic syndrome
F33.2		Recurrent depressive disorder, current episode severe without psychotic symptoms
F33.3		Recurrent depressive disorder, current episode severe with psychotic symptoms
	*.30	With mood-congruent psychotic symptoms
	*.31	With mood-incongruent psychotic symptoms
F33.4		Recurrent depressive disorder, currently in remission

F33.8	Other recurrent depressive disorders
F33.9	Recurrent depressive disorder, unspecified

F34 Persistent mood [affective] disorders

F34.0	Cyclothymia
F34.1	Dysthymia
F34.8	Other persistent mood [affective] disorders
F34.9	Persistent mood [affective] disorder, unspecified

F38 Other mood [affective] disorders

F38.0		Other single mood [affective] disorders
	.00	Mixed affective episode
F38.1		Other recurrent mood [affective] disorders
	.10	Recurrent brief depressive disorders
F38.8		Other specified mood [affective] disorders

F39 Unspecified mood [affective] disorder

F40–F48
Neurotic, stress-related and somatoform disorders

F40 Phobic anxiety disorders

F40.0		Agoraphobia
	.00	Without panic disorder
	.01	With panic disorder
F40.1		Social phobias
F40.2		Specific (isolated) phobias
F40.8		Other phobic anxiety disorders
F40.9		Phobic anxiety disorder, unspecified

F41 Other anxiety disorders

F41.0		Panic disorder [episodic paroxysmal anxiety]
	*.00	Moderate
	*.01	Severe

F41.1 Generalized anxiety disorder
F41.2 Mixed anxiety and depressive disorder
F41.3 Other mixed anxiety disorders
F41.8 Other specified anxiety disorders
F41.9 Anxiety disorder, unspecified

F42 Obsessive-compulsive disorder
F42.0 Predominantly obsessional thoughts or ruminations
F42.1 Predominantly compulsive acts [obsessional rituals]
F42.2 Mixed obsessional thoughts and acts
F42.8 Other obsessive–compulsive disorders
F42.9 Obsessive–compulsive disorder, unspecified

F43 Reaction to severe stress, and adjustment disorders
F43.0 Acute stress reaction
 *.00 Mild
 *.01 Moderate
 *.02 Severe
F43.1 Post-traumatic stress disorder
F43.2 Adjustment disorders
 .20 Brief depressive reaction
 .21 Prolonged depressive reaction
 .22 Mixed anxiety and depressive reaction
 .23 With predominant disturbance of other emotions
 .24 With predominant disturbance of conduct
 .25 With mixed disturbance of emotions and conduct
 .28 With other specified predominant symptoms
F43.8 Other reactions to severe stress

F43.9 Reaction to severe stress, unspecified

F44 Dissociative [conversion] disorders
F44.0 Dissociative amnesia
F44.1 Dissociative fugue
F44.2 Dissociative stupor
F44.3 Trance and possession disorders
F44.4 Dissociative motor disorders
F44.5 Dissociative convulsions
F44.6 Dissociative anaesthesia and sensory loss
F44.7 Mixed dissociative [conversion] disorders
F44.8 Other dissociative [conversion] disorders
 .80 Ganser's syndome
 .81 Multiple personality disorder
 .82 Transient dissociative [conversion] disorders occurring in childhood and adolescence
 .88 Other specified dissociative [conversion] disorders
F44.9 Dissociative [conversion] disorder, unspecified

F45 Somatoform disorders
F45.0 Somatization disorder
F45.1 Undifferentiated somatoform disorder
F45.2 Hypochondrial disorders
F45.3 Somatoform autonomic dysfunction
 .30 Heart and cardiovascular system
 .31 Upper gastrointestinal tract
 .32 Lower gastrointestinal tract
 .33 Respiratory system
 .34 Genitourinary system
 .38 Other organ or system
F45.4 Persistent somatoform pain disorder

| F45.8 | Other somatoform disorders |
| F45.9 | Somatoform disorder, unspecified |

F48 Other neurotic disorders

F48.0	Neurasthenia
F48.1	Depersonalization–derealization syndrome
F48.8	Other specified neurotic disorders
F48.9	Neurotic disorder, unspecified

F50–F59
Behavioural syndromes associated with physiological disturbances and physical factors

F50 Eating disorders

F50.0	Anorexia nervosa
F50.1	Atypical anorexia nervosa
F50.2	Bulimia nervosa
F50.3	Atypical bulimia nervosa
F50.4	Overeating associated with other psychological disturbances
F50.5	Vomiting associated with other psychological disturbances
F50.8	Other eating disorders
F50.9	Eating disorder, unspecified

F51 Non-organic sleep disorders

F51.0	Non-organic insomnia
F51.1	Non-organic hypersomnia
F51.2	Non-organic disorder of the sleep–wake schedule
F51.3	Sleepwalking [somnambulism]
F51.4	Sleep terrors [night terrors]
F51.5	Nightmares
F51.8	Other non-organic sleep disorders
F51.9	Non-organic sleep disorder, unspecified

F52 Sexual dysfunction, not caused by organic disorder or disease

F52.0	Lack or loss of sexual desire
F52.1	Sexual aversion and lack of sexual enjoyment
.10	Sexual aversion
.11	Lack of sexual enjoyment
F52.2	Failure of genital response
F52.3	Orgasmic dysfunction
F52.4	Premature ejaculation
F52.5	Non-organic vaginismus
F52.6	Non-organic dyspareunia
F52.7	Excessive sexual drive
F52.8	Other sexual dysfunction, not caused by organic disorder or disease
F52.9	Unspecified sexual dysfunction, not caused by organic disorder or disease

F53 Mental and behavioural disorders associated with the puerperium, not elsewhere classified

F53.0	Mild mental and behavioural disorders associated with the puerperium, not elsewhere classified
F53.1	Severe mental and behavioural disorders associated with the puerperium, not elsewhere classified
F53.8	Other mental and behavioural disorders associated with the puerperium, not elsewhere classified
F53.9	Puerperal mental disorder, unspecified

F54 Psychological and behavioural factors associated with disorders or diseases classified elsewhere

F55 Abuse of non-dependence-producing substances

F55.0	Antidepressants
F55.1	Laxatives
F55.2	Analgesics

F55.3	Antacids
F55.4	Vitamins
F55.5	Steroids or hormones
F55.6	Specific herbal or folk remedies
F55.8	Other substances that do not produce dependence
F55.9	Unspecified

F59 Unspecified behavioural syndromes associated with physiological disturbances and physical factors

F60–69
Disorders of adult personality and behaviour

F60 Specific personality disorders

F60.0	Paranoid personality disorder
F60.1	Schizoid personality disorder
F60.2	Dissocial personality disorder
F60.3	Emotionally unstable personality disorder
	.30 Impulsive type
	.31 Borderline type
F60.4	Histrionic personality disorder
F60.5	Anankastic personality disorder
F60.6	Anxious [avoidant] personality disorder
F60.7	Dependent personality disorder
F60.8	Other specific personality disorders
F60.9	Personality disorder, unspecified

F61 Mixed and other personality disorders

| F61.0 | Mixed personality disorder |
| F61.1 | Troublesome personality changes |

F62 Enduring personality changes, not attributable to brain damage and disease

F62.0	Enduring personality change after catastrophic experience
F62.1	Enduring personality change after psychiatric illness
F62.8	Other enduring personality changes
F62.9	Enduring personality change, unspecified

F63 Habit and impulse disorders

F63.0	Pathological gambling
F63.1	Pathological fire-setting [pyromania]
F63.2	Pathological stealing [kleptomania]
F63.3	Trichotillomania
F63.8	Other habit and impulse disorders
F63.9	Habit and impulse disorder, unspecified

F64 Gender identity disorders

F64.0	Transsexualism
F64.1	Dual-role transvestism
F64.2	Gender identity disorder of childhood
F64.8	Other gender identity disorders
F64.9	Gender identity disorders, unspecified

F65 Disorders of sexual preference

F65.0	Fetishism
F65.1	Fetishistic transvestism
F65.2	Exhibitionism
F65.3	Voyeurism
F65.4	Paedophilia
F65.5	Sadomasochism
F65.6	Multiple disorders of sexual preference
F65.8	Other disorders of sexual preference
F65.9	Disorder of sexual preference, unspecified

F66 Psychological and behavioural disorders

associated with sexual development and orientation

F66.0	Sexual maturation disorder
F66.1	Egodystonic sexual orientation
F66.2	Sexual relationship disorder
F66.8	Other psychosexual development disorders
F66.9	Psychosexual development disorder, unspecified

A fifth character may be used to indicate association with:

.x0	Heterosexuality
.x1	Homosexuality
.x2	Bisexuality
.x8	Other, including prepubertal

F68   Other disorders of adult personality and behaviour

F68.0	Elaboration of physical symptoms for psychological reasons
F68.1	Intentional production of feigning of symptoms or disabilities, either physical or psychological [factitious disorder]
F68.8	Other specified disorders of adult personality and behaviour
F69	**Unspecified disorder of adult personality and behaviour**

F70–F79
Mental retardation

F70	**Mild mental retardation**
F71	**Moderate mental retardation**
F72	**Severe mental retardation**
F73	**Profound mental retardation**
F78	**Other mental retardation**

F79   Unspecified mental retardation

A fourth character may be used to specify the extent of associated impairment of behaviour:

F7x.0	No, or minimal, impairment of behaviour
F7x.1	Significant impairment of behaviour requiring attention or treatment
F7x.2	Other impairments of behaviour
F7x.3	Without mention of impairment of behaviour

F80–F89
Disorders of psychological development

F80   Specific developmental disorders of speech and language

F80.0	Specific speech articulation disorder
F80.1	Expressive language disorder
F80.2	Receptive language disorder
F80.3	Acquired aphasia with epilepsy (Landau–Kleffner syndrome)
F80.8	Other developmental disorders of speech and language
F80.9	Development disorder of speech and language, unspecified

F81   Specific developmental disorders of scholastic skills

F81.0	Specific reading disorder
F81.1	Specific spelling disorder
F81.2	Specific disorder of arithmetical skills
F81.3	Mixed disorder of scholastic skills
F81.8	Other developmental disorders of scholastic skills

F81.9	Developmental disorder of scholastic skills, unspecified

F82 Specific development disorder of motor function

F83 Mixed specific developmental disorder

F84 Pervasive developmental disorders
F84.0	Childhood autism
F84.1	A typical autism
	*.10 Atypicality in age of onset
	*.11 Atypicality in symptomatology
	*.12 Atypicality in both age of onset and symptomatology
F84.2	Rett's syndrome
F84.3	Other childhood disintegrative disorder
F84.4	Overactive disorder associated with mental retardation and stereotyped movements
F84.5	Asperger's syndrome
F84.8	Other pervasive developmental disorders
F84.9	Pervasive developmental disorder, unspecified

F88 Other disorders of psychological development

F89 Unspecified disorder of psychological development

**F90–F98
Behavioural and emotional disorders with onset usually occurring in childhood and adolescence**

F90 Hyperkinetic disorder
F90.0	Disturbance of activity and attention
F90.1	Hyperkinetic conduct disorder
F90.8	Other hyperkinetic disorders

F90.9	Hyperkinetic disorder, unspecified

F91 Conduct disorders
F91.0	Conduct disorder confined to the family context
F91.1	Unsocialized conduct disorder
F91.2	Socialized conduct disorder
F91.3	Oppositional defiant disorder
F91.8	Other conduct disorders
F91.9	Conduct disorder, unspecified

F92 Mixed disorders of conduct and emotions
F92.0	Depressive conduct disorder
F92.8	Other mixed disorders of conduct and emotions
F92.9	Mixed disorder of conduct and emotions, unspecified

F93 Emotional disorders with onset specific to childhood
F93.0	Separation anxiety disorder of childhood
F93.1	Phobic anxiety disorder of childhood
F93.2	Social anxiety disorder of childhood
F93.3	Sibling rivalry disorder
F93.8	Other childhood emotional disorders
	*.80 Generalized anxiety disorder of childhood
F93.9	Childhood emotional disorder, unspecified

F94 Disorders of social functioning with onset specific to childhood and adolescence
F94.0	Elective mutism
F94.1	Reactive attachment disorder of childhood
F94.2	Disinhibited attachment disorder of childhood
F94.8	Other childhood disorders of social functioning

F94.9 Childhood disorder of social functioning, unspecified

F95 Tic disorders
F95.0 Transient tic disorders
F95.1 Chronic motor or vocal tic disorder
F95.2 Combined vocal and multiple motor tic disorder [de la Tourette's syndrome]
F95.8 Other tic disorders
F95.8 Tic disorder, unspecified

F98 Other behavioural and emotional disorders with onset usually occurring in childhood and adolescence
F98.0 Non-organic enuresis
   *.00 Nocturnal enuresis only
   *.01 Diurnal enuresis only
   *.02 Nocturnal and diurnal enureses
F98.1 Non-organic encopresis
   *.10 Failure to acquire physiological bowel control
   *.11 Adequate bowel control with normal faeces deposited in inappropriate places
   *.12 Soiling that is associated with excessively fluid faeces, such as with retention with overflow
F98.2 Feeding disorder of infancy and childhood
F98.3 Pica of infancy and childhood
F98.4 Stereotyped movement disorders
   *.40 Non-self-injurious
   *.41 Self-injurious
   *.42 Mixed
F98.5 Stuttering [stammering]
F98.6 Cluttering
F98.8 Other specified behavioural and emotional disorders with onset usually occurring in childhood and adolescence
F98.9 Unspecified behavioural and emotional disorders with onset usually occurring in childhood and adolescence

F99
Unspecified mental disorder

F99 Mental disorder not otherwise specified

Appendix 8
Glossary of key features of ICD-10 personality disorder categories

The following is a summary of the key features of the ICD-10 personality disorder categories: the number in parentheses indicates the number of attributes that should be present for **abnormality of personality** of that type to be confidently diagnosed; the presence of distress or handicap, in addition, makes the diagnosis one of **personality disorder**.

Paranoid (4)
Sensitivity to rebuff, sensitive to own rights, bears grudges, suspicious, self-important, self-referential, conspiratorial view of the world.

Schizoid (4)
Little pleasure in ordinary activities, cold, doesn't show affection, indifferent to others' opinions, prefers solitary pastimes, disinterested in friendship, disregard for social norms, excessively introspective.

Dissocial (3)
Callous unconcern for others' feelings, persistent irresponsibility, can't keep relationships, low tolerance for frustration, low threshold for aggression, doesn't feel guilty, blames others for own behaviours that have caused conflict.

Emotionally unstable — impulsive (3)
Quarrelsome*, acts unexpectedly, outbursts of anger, difficulty in sustaining activity, unstable mood.   (*Mandatory)

Emotionally unstable — borderline
Should show most of 'impulsive' features as above; plus *two* of the following:- uncertainty about self-image and aims in life; easily and intensively involved in relationships; fear of abandonment; threats of self-harm; feeling of emptiness.

Histrionic (4)
Theatrical, suggestible, shallow affect, seeks excitement, likes to be the centre of attention, over concerned about physical attractiveness, inappropriately seductive.

Anankastic (4)

Excessive doubt or caution, preoccupation with details or rules, perfectionist, excessively conscientious, over concern with task in hand to the exclusion of pleasure, pedantic, rigid or stubborn, unreasonable insistence on others doing things his/her way.

Anxious/Avoidant (4)

Persistent apprehension, strong sense of being socially inept or inferior, preoccupied with criticisms/rejection in social circumstances, cautious of involvement, restricted life style for reasons of security, avoidance of circumstances that might lead to criticism/dissaproval from others.

Dependent (4)

Wants others to make decisions, unduly complacent, doesn't make even reasonable demands on others, uncomfortable/anxious when alone, preoccupied with fears of having to manage alone, needs advice/reassurance on day-to-day decisions.

Index